1495 D

18/70 H
less 20%

EAR ACUPRESSURE

A layman's guide to the therapeutic use of finger pressure on the acupuncture points of the ear

By the same author:
ELECTRO-ACUPUNCTURE:
Its Clinical Applications in Therapy

EAR ACUPRESSURE

The Ancient Chinese Art of Healing and Treating Pain with Finger Pressure

by

PEDRO CHAN

THORSONS

THORSONS PUBLISHERS LIMITED
Wellingborough, Northamptonshire

First published in the United Kingdom 1981

Original American edition published by Chan's Corporation, Monterey Park, California.

British Library Cataloguing in Publication Data

Chan, Pedro
Ear acupressure
1. Acupressure
2. Ear
I. Title
615.8'22 RM723.A27

ISBN 0-7225-0727-5

Printed in Great Britain by
The Thetford Press Limited, Thetford, Norfolk,
and bound by Weatherby Woolnough,
Wellingborough, Northamptonshire.

NOTE

Ear acupressure is not a cure. It is also not the intention of the author to provide a substitute for medical diagnosis, acupuncture or conventional Western therapy. Finger ear acupressure should be used as a supplement after determining the nature of the disorder.

Dedicated to Bart

CONTENTS

FOREWORD

Two historic visits to China by American Presidents and visits by leading American physicians and writers set the stage for a heightened interest in Chinese medicine, especially acupuncture. Through this interest, Western physicians, medical schools and lay public are beginning to discover many valuable therapeutic and prophylactic uses for this traditional medical art.

Let us consider research concerning acupuncture points in the ear. The ear has over 200 points, each of them having a specific relationship to an organ or area of the body. In particular, early research indicates that some of those points can be used effectively in treating compulsive disorders such as obesity, drug addiction, alcoholism, and smoking, and also for treating pain relating to other disorders. Ear acupressure (stimulation of points in the ear by massage) has gained favor as a new method for treating pain and these compulsive disorders because (1) it works, (2) it is easy to use, and (3) it can help patients without the harmful side effects of drugs.

Pedro Chan has the unique ability to present the difficult subject of ear acupressure in such a way that all can understand and apply it.

John F. Chow, Pharm. D., M.D.
Medical Director,
Center for Chinese Medicine

INTRODUCTION

All of us are aware that the ear is the organ of hearing, but few know that it is also the center for controlling equilibrium. And very few of us know that the ear represents an inverted miniature of the human embryo.

Anatomists divide the ear into three areas: (1) the external, (2) middle, and (3) inner ear. The external ear includes the auricle and the external auditory meatus (the ear canal). Most people refer to the auricle as being the "ear." This is the part of the ear that we are interested in studying in this book.

What Ear Acupuncture and Acupressure Is

Ear acupuncture is being used at leading medical schools and treatment centers in the United States, Canada, France, China and throughout the world to treat disorders such as obesity, smoking, low back pain, and headaches. This art of healing, which involves the insertion of needles into specific points of the ear, is called ear acupuncture. Ear acupressure is an innovative outgrowth of ear acupuncture. By substituting finger pressure over these specific points, it is called ear acupressure.

A Brief History

The ear is first mentioned in the earliest Chinese medical book, *Yellow Emperor's Classics of Internal Medicine*, published more than 2,000 years ago. It states that the ear is not independent but relates to all parts of the human body and internal organs. This can be considered the beginning of the utilization of the ear for medical/clinical purposes. Several books have mentioned the clinical applications that utilize the ear. Even today, among those familiar with Chinese tradition, it is fairly well-known that pulling the ear lobes can relieve headaches; squeezing the ear lobes can treat children's convulsions. These are just two examples which demonstrate the early use of ear acupressure in Chinese traditional medicine.

Development Today

Knowledge about ear acupuncture has been well researched and documented. In 1956, the Chinese reported using ear acupuncture to treat throat numbness. In 1957, Dr. Paul Nogier, a well-known French neurosurgeon, made a careful study of the ear and its relationship to the rest of the body. He has developed the French "Auricular Therapy," which is based on his neuro-embryal theory.

Currently, there are more than 200 points which have been discovered in the ear. This is mainly the result of accumulated research work in China during the past 10 years.

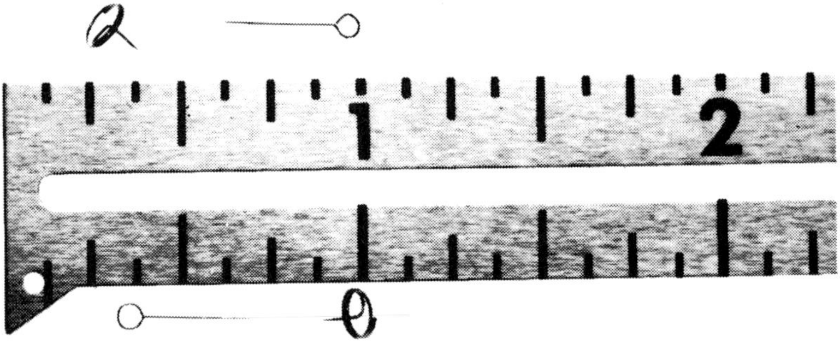

Press needles and Interdermal needles (with longer needle body).

The most commonly used type of stimulation of ear acupuncture points is needle insertion. For ear use, there are several types of needles: (1) regular half-inch and one-inch, (2) press needles, and (3) interdermal needles. The latter two types of needles are imbedded into the skin and left in place with a piece of tape covering the area. The needles are imbedded in order to provide continuous stimulation. However, the needles do not always remain imbedded. Lester Sacks, M.D., of Torrance, California, realized this problem and solved it by using a surgical staple in the ear. It is called Staple-puncture. A similar technique is to suture beads in the ear. There is still another way of providing continuous stimulation – by taping a minute ion steel ball on an adhesive patch over the ear acupuncture point. These are called ion patches in Japan and "Acu-aid" in America.

There are other modalities used in ear therapy. These include Sono-puncture, which provides ultra-sound stimulation over ear points. This medical electronic instrument has a specially designed transducer head, only one to two millimeters in diameter. It is called Khoe's head, named after its inventor, Willem Khoe, M.D., a prominent medical acupuncturist in Sun Valley, California.

Another modality is aqua-puncture. It requires the injection of a particular fluid into ear points. Distilled water, saline, Vitamins B_1 and B_{12} are often used.

Moxibustion involves the application of thermal (heat) stimulation. Many traditional practitioners prefer using the herb wormwood rather than electrical heat, ultra-violet rays, or infra-red rays because of its beneficial penetrating heat.

The most beneficial ear stimulation in my experience is the use of electrical treatment. This occurs by passing electrical current into two specific points through needles or surface electrodes. Using electricity with needles is called Electro-acupuncture. The use of electricity with surface electrodes is called Transcutaneous Nerve Stimulation.

The safest and most economical means of stimulation, however, is finger pressure. At one time, the author attended an auricular acupuncture seminar at which the famous French authority, Dr. Rene Bourdiol, was the main speaker. He said that he is using more and more finger pressure massage rather than needles, because it works as well as the needle.

Clinical Applications

There are at least four major applications of ear acupuncture or acupressure: (1) preventive medicine, (2) therapy, (3) diagnostic aid, and (4) surgical analgesia. In China, many operations have been performed while patients were under ear acupuncture analgesia. However, this is not within our scope of discussion in this book.

Ear acupuncture as a preventive medicine is still under investigation. Preliminary success has been found in preventing malaria, motion sickness and recurrence of asthma.

For diagnostic purposes, one or more responsive points are sought. Under normal conditions, the ear points of a healthy person do not have any special responses. When a problem exists in an internal organ(s) or any other part(s) of the body, there are one or more responsive ear points corresponding to the disorder. Generally, the number of points which respond is directly proportional to the intensity of the illness. However, the point(s) can only reflect the area(s) and/or organ(s) of the disorder. It does not indicate the cause of the disorder. A Chinese study reported that fracture of the leg in monkeys or rabbits causes some points to respond in the ear's Triangular Fossa and Antihelix. These two areas of the ear represent pain and the leg area. In another study of 288 TB patients in one hospital, 286 of them showed responses to a point in the Lung area of the ear.

This book mainly discusses the therapeutic aspect of ear acupressure and its use by the layman. First, let us examine some important statistics regarding ear acupuncture. Ear acupuncture can treat as many disorders as "body" acupuncture can. In thousands of cases treated with ear acupuncture in China, efficacy has proven 70 to 80 percent. In many cases, it has proven over 90 percent effective. Examples of most successful treatments include nausea, vomiting, stomach spasm, diarrhea, enteritis, indigestion, constipation, alcoholism, smoking (nicotine addiction), chest pain, headaches, heat stroke, malaria, sprains, painful menstruation, Meniere syndromes, toothache, etc.

Ear acupressure is not a cure. There are no panaceas. It is also not the intention of the author to provide a substitute for medical diagnosis, acupuncture or conventional Western therapy. Finger ear acupressure should be used only after determining the nature of the disorder. If the condition persists, be sure to see a licensed physician.

ORGANIZATION OF THE EAR

The ear is made up of a thin layer of skin covering a thin irregular plate structure of elastic cartilage. There is no cartilage in the lobe.

ANATOMY AND PHYSIOLOGY OF THE EAR IN ACUPUNCTURE AND ACUPRESSURE

Descriptively, the ear is thought to simulate an inverted fetus within the womb.

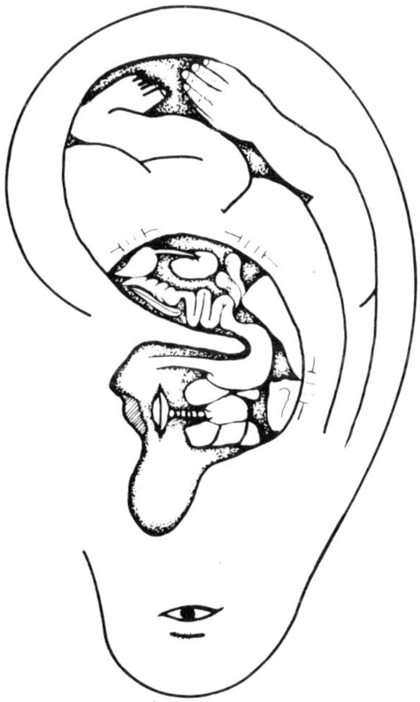

Descriptively, the ear is thought to simulate an inverted fetus within the womb (front). (Courtesy of Chan's Corporation, Alhambra, CA)

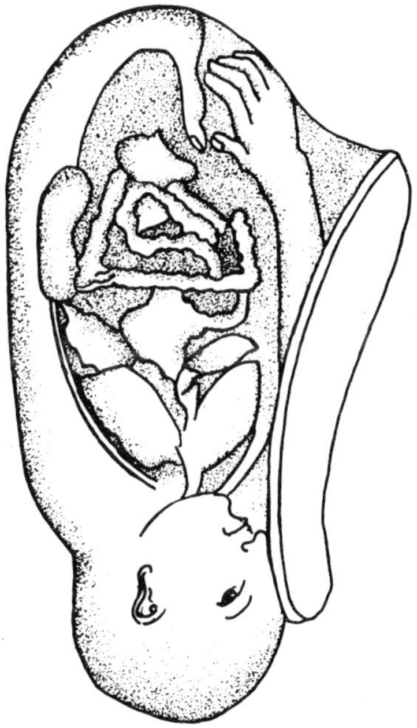

Descriptively, the ear is thought to simulate an inverted fetus within the womb (back). (Courtesy of Chan's Corporation, Alhambra, CA)

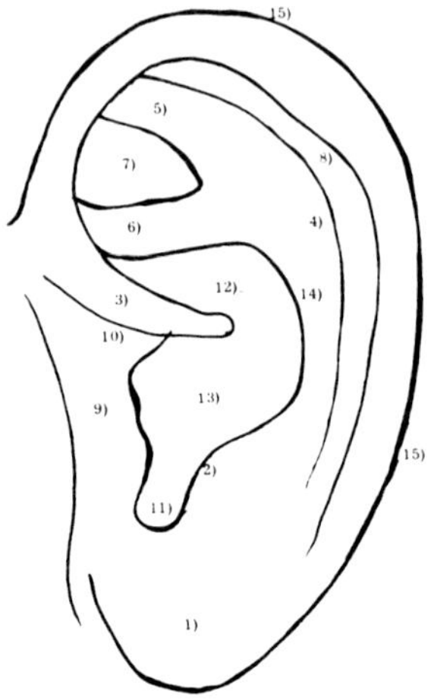

1. Lobe
2. Antitragus
3. Helix Limb
4. Antihelix
5. Upper Limb of Antihelix
6. Lower Limb of Antihelix
7. Triangular Fossa
8. Scapha
9. Tragus
10. Supratragic Notch
11. Intertragic Notch
12. Cymba Concha
13. Cavum Concha
14. Concha Edge of Antihelix
15. Helix

Anatomy and physiology of the ear in Acupuncture or Acupressure

1. Lobe

Anatomy: Lower portion of ear.
Acu-designation: Corresponds to facial region.

2. Antitragus

Anatomy: An elevation above the lobe.
Acu-designation: Corresponds to head region.

3. Helix Limb

Anatomy: Transverse portion of Helix extending into Concha.
Acu-designation: Corresponds to diaphragm.
Region around the Helix Limb corresponds to digestive tract.

4. Antihelix

Anatomy: Curved ridge in front of Helix.
Acu-designation: Corresponds to trunk.

5. Upper Limb of Antihelix

Anatomy: Upward branch of Antihelix.
Acu-designation: Corresponds to lower extremities.

6. Lower Limb of Antihelix

Anatomy: Downward branch of Antihelix.
Acu-designation: Corresponds to buttocks.

7. Triangular Fossa

Anatomy: Triangular depression between Upper and Lower Limbs of Antihelix.
Acu-designation: Corresponds to genital organs.

8. Scapha

Anatomy: Bow-shaped groove between Helix and Antihelix.
Acu-designation: Corresponds to upper extremities.

9. Tragus

Anatomy: The fleshy protrusion in front of ear.

10. Supratragic Notch

Anatomy: Depressed part between upper Tragus and Limb of Helix.

11. Intertragic Notch

Anatomy: In depression between lower Tragus and Antitragus.
Acu-designation: Corresponds to internal secretion.

12. Cymba Concha

Anatomy: Portion of Concha above Limb of Helix.
Acu-designation: Corresponds to abdominal region.

13. Cavum Concha

Anatomy: Portion of Concha below Limb of Helix.
Acu-designation: Corresponds to chest region.

Ear model showing areas of inverted fetus as theorized in ear acupuncture

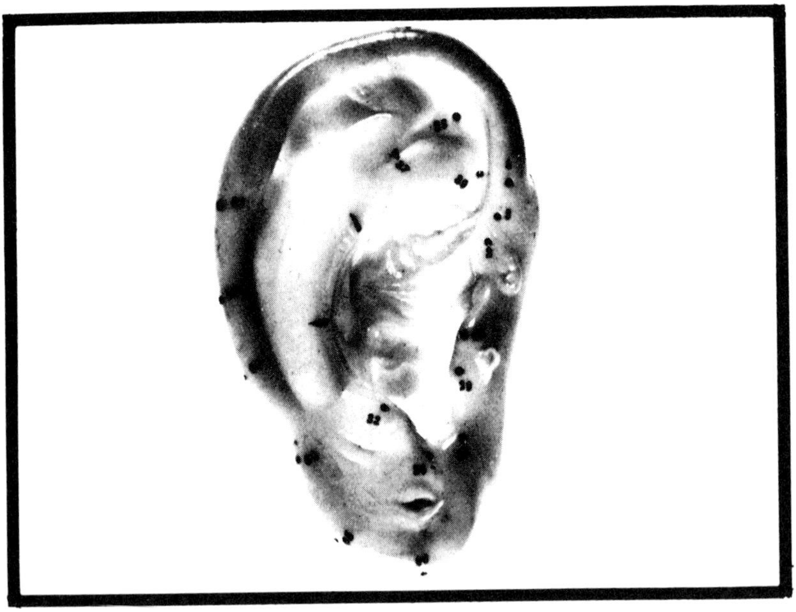

14. Concha Edge of Antihelix

Anatomy: Curved edge of the Antihelix with Concha.
Acu-designation: Corresponds to spinal column.

15. Helix

Anatomy: Outer curved rim of ear.

16. Back of Ear

Anatomy: At the back of the ear.
Acu-designation: Corresponds to back region of fetus.

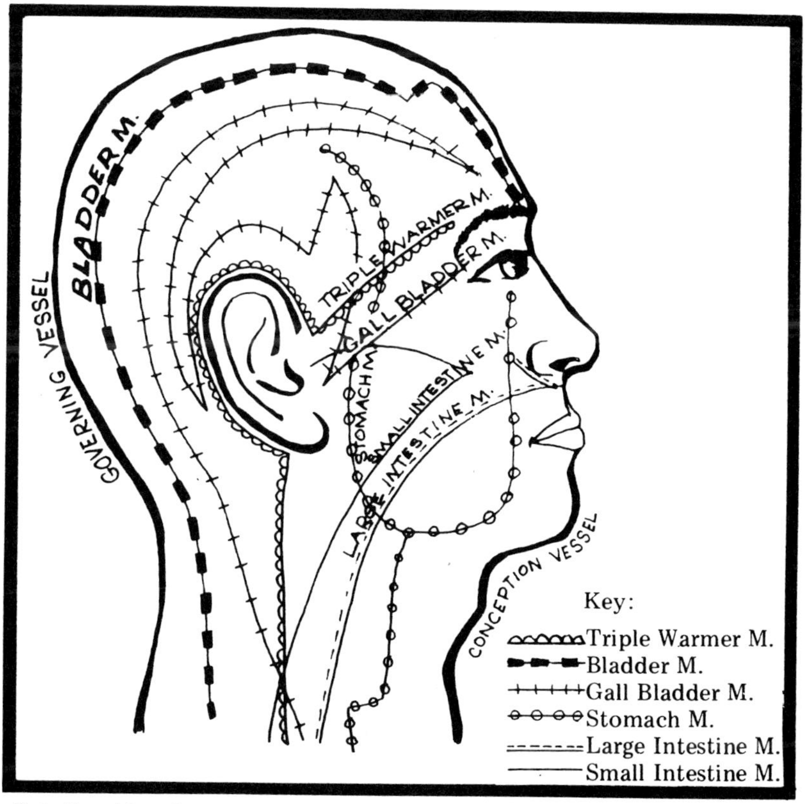

Relationship of Acupuncture Meridians to the Ear

RELATIONSHIP OF ACUPUNCTURE MERIDIANS TO THE EAR

The pathways of six main acupuncture meridians run directly by or close to the ear. They are the Large Intestine, Stomach, Small Intestine, Bladder, Triple Warmer, and Gall Bladder meridians. These belong to the Yang meridians (see following table). You can now see that the ear is directly or indirectly related to the 12 main pairs of meridians which run over the body.

YANG MERIDIANS	YIN MERIDIANS
Large Intestine	Lung
Stomach	Spleen
Small Intestine	Heart
Bladder	Kidney
Triple Warmer	Pericardium
Gall Bladder	Liver

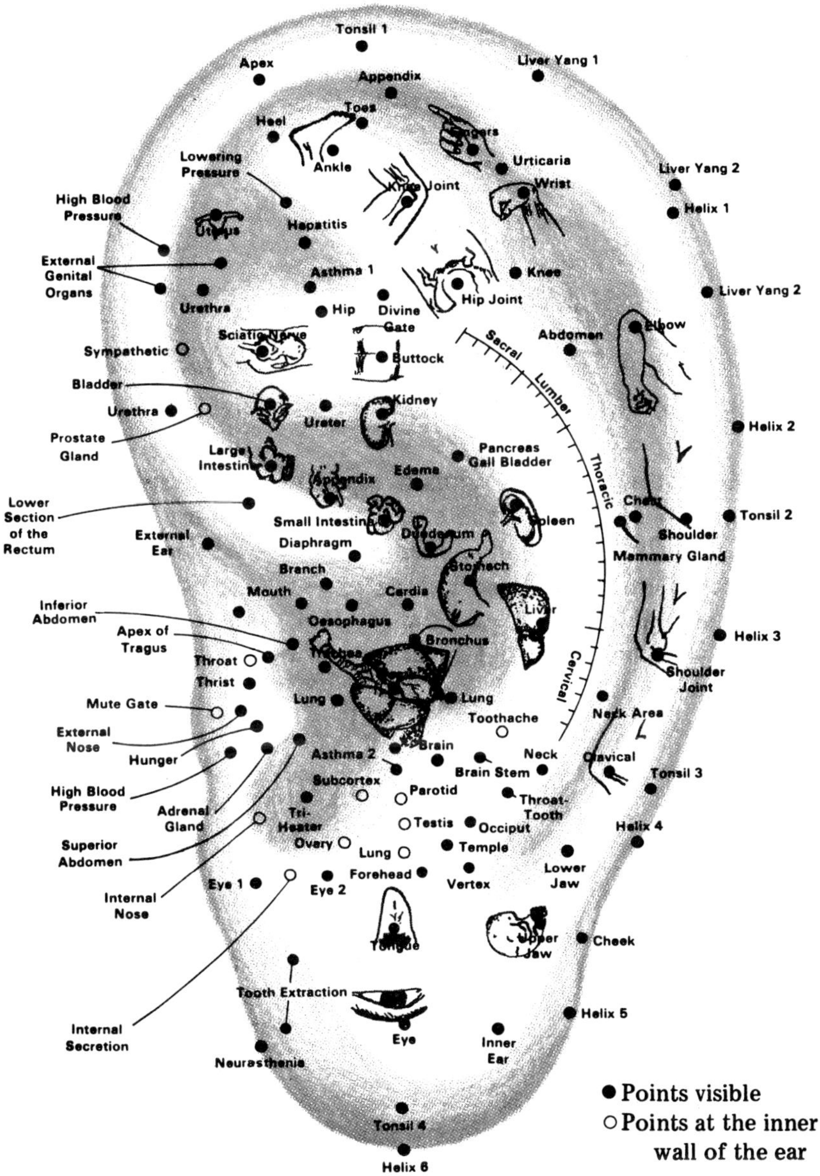

Distribution of Ear Points (courtesy of Chan's Corporation, Alhambra, CA)

DISTRIBUTION OF EAR POINTS

Important therapeutic points related to specific disorders are described here. These points are arranged in alphabetical order. For exact location, refer to *Locating the Ear Acupressure Point* under *Essentials of Ear Acupressure* in the next chapter.

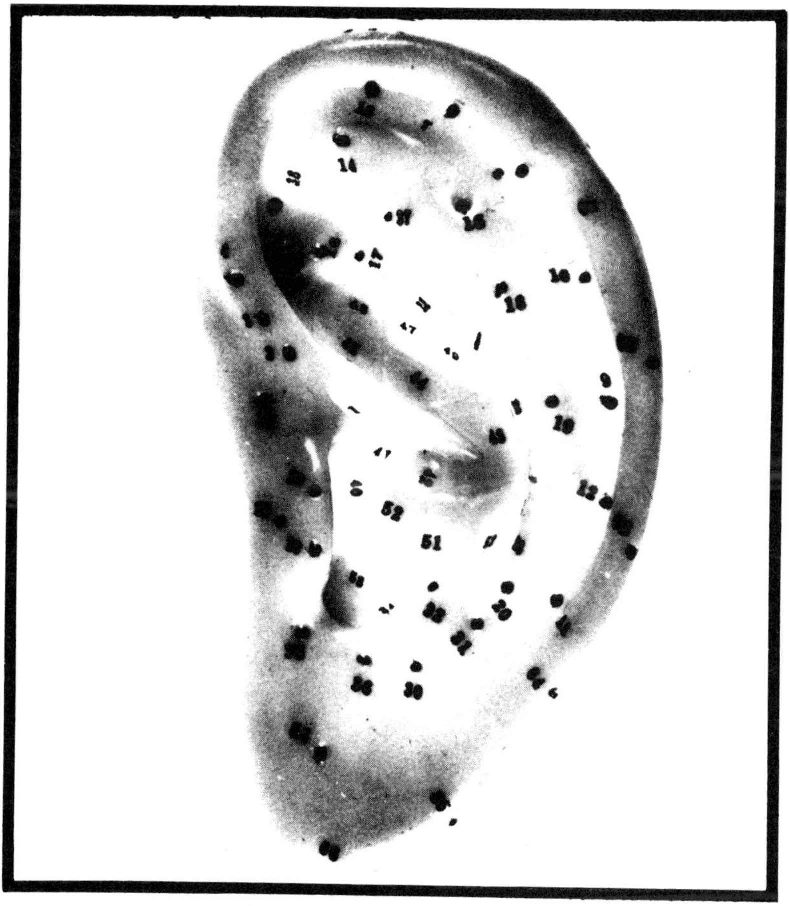

Points on ear model from China

Abdomen

Location: On the antihelix, and on the same level with the Lower Limb of the Antihelix.

Indications: Spasmodic pain of internal organs (stomach, intestines, etc.).

Adrenal Gland

Location: At the edge of lower part of Tragus.

Indications: Hypertension, hypotension, fever, inflammation, rheumatism and skin disorders.

Ankle

Location: At the inner corner of Upper Limb of Antihelix.

Indications: Pain or functional disorders of ankle.

Bladder

Location: In the Cymba Concha, close to the Lower Limb of Antihelix.

Indications: Cystitis (inflammation of bladder), retention of urine, enuresis (bedwetting) and lumbago (low back pain).

Chest

Location: On the Antihelix, at the same level with Supratragic Notch.

Indications: Intercostal (rib) pain, chest congestion.

Diaphragm

Location: On the Limb of the Helix.

Indications: Spasms of the diaphragm muscle, itching, skin disorders, nosebleed.

Divine Gate

Location: At the meeting point of the Lower and Upper Limbs of Antihelix.

Indications: Pain, inflammation, nervousness, and itching.

Elbow

Location: In the Scapha, between Wrist and Shoulder.
Indications: Pain or functional disorders of elbow.

External Genital Organs

Location: On the Helix, at the level of Lower Limb of Antihelix.
Indications: Impotence, eczema of scrotum, low back pain, Sciatica.

Eye

Location: At the center of the ear Lobe.
Indications: Eye disorders.

Finger

Location: At the upper part of the Scapha.
Indications: Pain or functional disorders of finger.

Forehead

Location: Just below the Antitragus.
Indications: Sinusitis, toothache, and giddiness.

Gall Bladder

Location: In the Cymba Concha, on the right side of the Kidney.
Indications: Cholecystitis (inflammation of gall bladder), gallstones, worms.

Heart

Location: In the center of Cavum Concha.
Indications: Dreaminess, insomnia, glossitis (inflammation of tongue), anemia.

Hunger

Location: Just below the center point of the front Tragus.
Indications: Hunger, diabetes.

Internal Secretion

Location: In the Cavum Concha, behind the Intertragic Notch.
Indications: Functional disorders of internal secretion, and skin diseases. Often used for female diseases, urogenital disorders.

Kidney

Location: In the Cymba Concha, at the lower part of Lower Limb of Antihelix.
Indications: Nerve deafness, tinnitus (ringing in the ears), decreasing hearing, eye disorders, female disorders, urinary disorders, pain caused by bone fractures, hair loss, baldness, loss of memory, tiredness, edema, impotence, and loose teeth.

Knee

Location: On the Antihelix, at the level of the meeting point of Lower and Upper Limbs of Antihelix.
Indications: Pain or functional disorders of the knee.

Large Intestine

Location: In the Cymba Concha, above the Limb of Antihelix.
Indications: Dysentery, enteritis (inflammation of intestinal tract), diarrhea, constipation, and hemorrhoids.

Liver

Location: In the Cymba Concha, below the Spleen.
Indications: Hepatitis (inflammation of liver), eye disorders,

disorders associated with the blood, rheumatism, iron-deficient anemia, neuralgia, headache, dizziness.

Lumbo-Sacral, Thoracic, and Cervical Vertebrae

Location: On the Concha edge of the Antihelix. From above downward: first part includes the lumbo-sacral vertebrae; second, by the thoracic vertebrae; and the third, the cervical vertebrae.

Indications: Corresponding vertebral pain or functional disorders.

Lung

Location: In the Cavum Concha, surrounding the Heart.

Indications: Diseases of the respiratory system, skin disorders, loss of hair, and rhinitis (inflammation of nose).

Mouth

Location: In the Cavum Concha, near the opening of external auditory canal.

Indications: Ulcer of mouth, glossitis (inflammation of tongue) and lock-jaw.

Neck

Location: At the junction of the Antihelix and Antitragus.

Indications: Pain or functional disorders.

Occiput

Location: On the side of the Antitragus.

Indications: Disorders of the nervous system, the respiratory system, the eye and the skin, and motion-sickness. Good also for relief of pain and inflammation.

Ovary

Location: At the lower part of the inner wall of the Antitragus. This is part of the Subcortex.
Indications: Frigidity, amenorrhea (irregular menses), dysmenorrhea (painful menstruation), sterility.

Pancreas

Location: In the Cymba Concha, at the right side of the Gall Bladder.
Indications: Pancreatitis (inflammation of pancreas), diabetes, dyspepsia (disturbed digestion).

Prostate Gland

Location: In the Cymba Concha, above the Bladder.
Indications: Prostatitis (inflammation of prostate), pain in urination, premature ejaculation, and spermatorrhea (involuntary discharge of semen without orgasm).

Sciatic Nerve

Location: On the midpoint of the Lower Limb of Antihelix, close to the Cymba Concha region.
Indications: Sciatica.

Shoulder

Location: In the Scapha, level with the Supratragic Notch.
Indications: Pain or functional disorders.

Small Intestine

Location: In the Cymba Concha, above the lower part of the Limb of Antihelix.
Indications: Dyspepsia (disturbed digestion), intestinal distension, duodenal ulcer, and heart disease.

Soothing Asthma

Location: At the top of Antitragus.
Indications: Cough, asthma, itching.

Spleen

Location: In the Cymba Concha, on the right side of the Stomach.
Indications: Indigestion, muscular atrophy, prolapse of rectum, weakness after sickness.

Stomach

Location: In the Cavum Concha, at the end of the Limb of Antihelix.
Indications: Disorders of digestive system, such as indigestion, ulcer, gastritis, swelling; also insomnia.

Subcortex

Location: In the inner wall of the Antitragus.
Indications: Pain, inflammation, nervousness, gastroptosis (prolapse or downward displacement of stomach), and hysperoptosis (falling or inversion of uterus).

Sympathetic Nerve

Location: In the Triangular Fossa, at junction of Lower Limb of Antihelix and Helix border.
Indications: Pain and spasm of internal organs, eye disorders, vascular inflammation.

Temple

Location: Behind the Antitragus, between Occiput and Forehead.

Indications: Dizziness, giddiness, sleeping sickness, and migraine headache.

Testis

Location: At the lower part of the inner wall of Antitragus. This is part of the Subcortex.
Indications: Impotence, orchitis (inflammation of testis).

Toe

Location: On the corner of the Upper Limb of Antihelix.
Indications: Pain or functional disorders of the toe.

Trachea

Location: In the Cavum Concha, between Heart and Lung.
Indications: Bronchitis, asthma.

Uterus

Location: On the Triangular Fossa, close to the border with the Helix.
Indications: Female disorders, male functional decrement (lessening of male function), and epididymitis (inflammation of seminal duct).

Vertex

Location: In the Lobe, below the Temple.
Indications: Vertical headache, dizziness.

Wrist

Location: In the Scapha, below the Finger.
Indications: Pain or functional disorders of the wrist.

ESSENTIALS OF EAR ACUPRESSURE

Posture

No matter what your partner's posture is — lying down, sitting up or standing — your partner must be relaxed, comfortable, and natural. You must be able to fully utilize your finger movement and strength.

Finger Pressure

The degree of pressure varies with the condition and physique of your partner. The author will go over the technique for each problem in treatment chapters. Anyway, if you are using pressure properly, your partner should feel numbness, soreness, heat, or coolness radiating from the point being massaged. These sensations may also appear over or around the diseased area, following certain pathways.

Manipulation

There are three ways of applying finger manipulation: (1) finger nail, (2) finger tip, and (3) finger flat. When applying

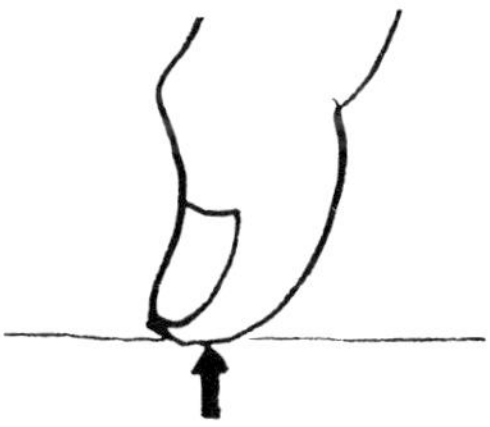

Finger tip pressure

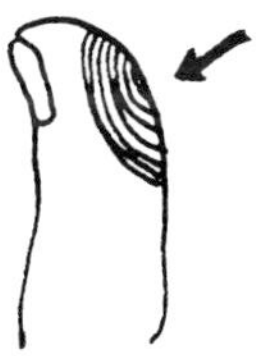

Finger flat pressure

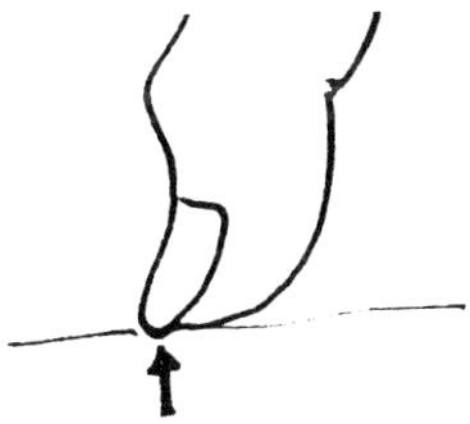

Finger nail pressure

finger nail or tip pressure, always keep finger vertical in relation to the designated point on the skin surface. Massage the point in small circular movements. Be careful to move only the finger, not the ear. The speed and degree of pressure play an important part in the effectiveness of manipulation. Their importance will be discussed for each individual treatment later.

The French ear pressure techniques are somewhat more sophisticated. When making the circular motion, if the finger is moving toward the center, it is called *tonification*, which means mild stimulation. If the finger moves away from the center, it is called *dispersion*, which means strong stimulation. The French often use a smooth and round-tipped glass rod instead of a finger. If you don't wish to use your finger and you do not have a glass rod, you may use any similar object which has a smooth and round-headed tip.

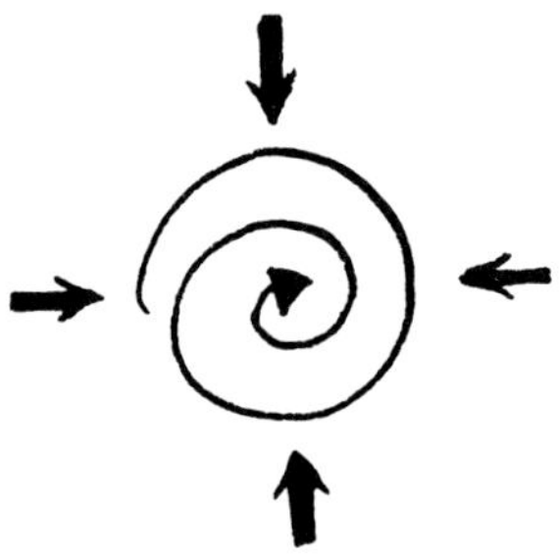

Massage toward the center is to give tonification. (Mild stimulation.)

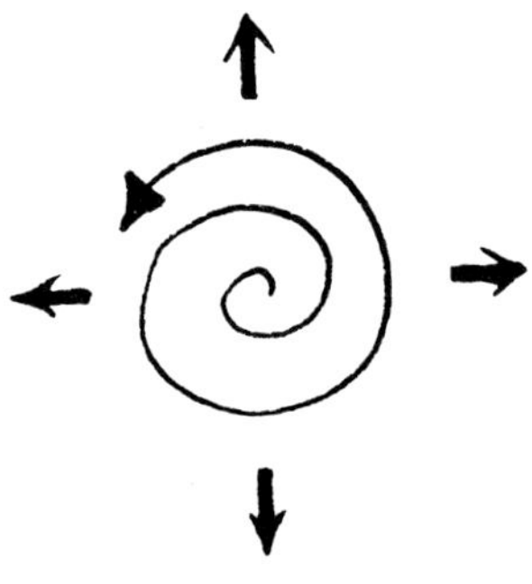

Massage away from the center is to give dispersion. (Strong stimulation.)

Period of Treatment

Finger massage is given in periods ranging from one to five minutes for each point per treatment. You may apply stimulation once daily or whenever you have symptoms. The author finds that often the best time to start treatment is just prior to symptom(s), or when one feels on the verge of having the symptom(s).

Locating the Ear Acupressure Point

Although each point is defined, exact location differs from person to person; it may change from condition to condition. There are certain ways of detecting the accurate location of an ear point. They are as follows:

1. Appearance: The ear point(s) related to the disorders may appear physically different from adjacent area in color and shape. It may look more yellowish, whitish, or pinkish. There may be slight swelling, peeling, or a small pimple.

2. Sensitivity: The point(s) may be more sensitive to pressure with respect to adjacent area(s). Sensitivity can be detected by gently touching the ear surface with constant, consistent pressure. If your partner responds to certain points with a greater degree of pain, those spots are considered the specific ear acupressure points to be used. The finger flat or a glass rod may be used for the pulsating. It is important to apply constant, consistent pressure to all areas for detecting proper ear points.

3. Response to Electrical Resistance: The point(s) may show lower electrical resistance with respect to the adjacent area. To perform this, an electronic instrument called a Point-finder or Punctoscope is required.

4. Skin Temperature: The point(s) may have a higher temperature than the adjacent area. There may be one or more degrees (F) difference. This is understandable since skin temperature is inversely proportional to electrical resistance of skin. To measure skin temperature of the ear, a special thermister is required.

The above methods can be used individually, in combination or all together. Practitioners make their own intelligent judgment regarding which type(s) to utilize.

Points may be located as described previously in both ears. Generally, the ear of the disorder's side is treated. If you are not sure, both ears should be treated. In either case, for every treatment and each ear, the same technique should be repeated.

There are some natural responsive points existing in the ear all the time. It is wise, therefore, to be very careful in distinguishing them when detecting the real responsive ear point.

Precaution

Always keep the following precautions in mind:

1. You should keep your hands, fingers, fingernails clean and warm. Fingernails should be trimmed just slightly beyond the skin tip of the finger. This provides a good grip for manipulation.

2. Never give ear acupressure to your partner if the person has a full or empty stomach. Treatment with exhausted or nervous patients is not recommended.

3. Ear acupressure is not to be applied during pregnancy or on serious cardiac patients.

4. Avoid working on skin surface of any contusion, scar, or infection of ear.

5. Massaging ear points is somewhat painful. It is not recommended for infants or very young children.

6. Stop treatment if symptom is aggravated or no relief is observed.

Diet

Diet plays an important role in Chinese medicine. Several cases are presented under treatment chapters.

What to Do if Ear Acupressure Doesn't Work

Generally speaking, results of finger pressure techniques are successful, but often slower and temporary compared to needle therapy (acupuncture). If you do not get results, try corresponding point(s) at the back of the ear, or a combination of ear and body points.

If you still have no results after three to four weeks, either you are not giving ear acupressure properly or you are not responding to the pressure treatment. In either case, consult your physician or acupuncturist.

A GUIDE TO EAR POINT SELECTION FOR DISORDERS IN VARIOUS SYSTEMS

The following ear points are listed for your reference only. They are general treatment points for disorders mentioned. Although a number of points are given, only those that reveal greatest response should be used. Always minimize the use of ear points to one or two in each ear, if possible.

DIGESTIVE SYSTEM

Example: Nausea, vomiting, gastritis (inflammation of stomach), stomach or duodenal ulcer, gastric spasm, gall bladder inflammation, pancreatitis (inflammation of pancreas), diarrhea, enteritis (inflammation of intestines), indigestion, intestinal colic (pain due to smooth muscle spasm).

Points: Stomach
Large Intestine
Small Intestine
Pancreas
Gall Bladder
Spleen
Liver
Sympathetic Nerve
Abdomen
Internal Secretion
Divine Gate

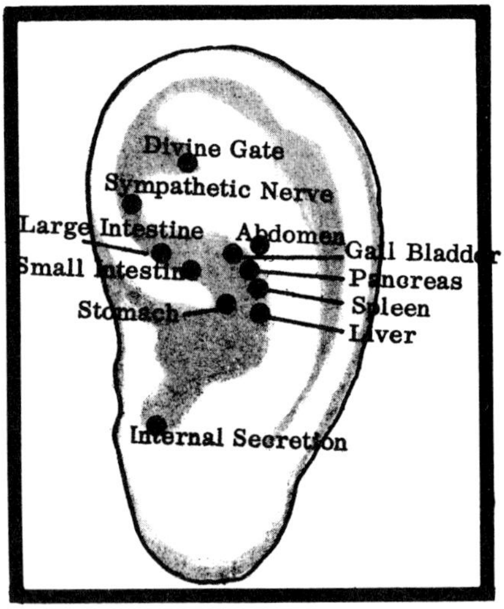

RESPIRATORY SYSTEM

Examples: Cough, chest pain, bronchitis (inflammation of mucous membrane of bronchi), asthma, whooping cough, pneumonia.

Points: Soothing Asthma
Trachea
Lung
Chest
Occiput
Divine Gate
Sympathetic Nerve
Internal Secretion

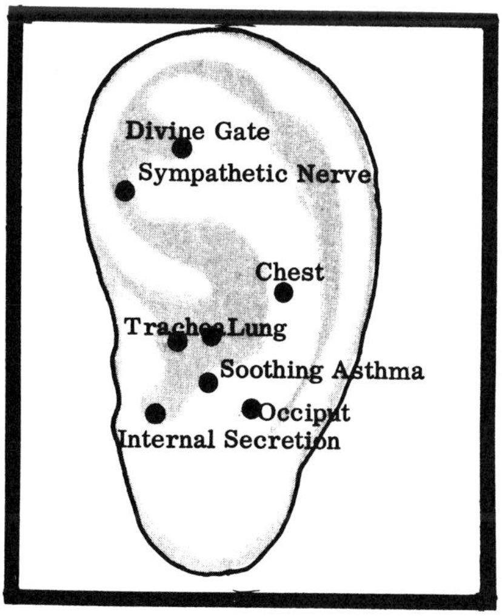

CIRCULATORY SYSTEM

Examples: Hypertension, hypotension, feeble pulse.

Points: Heart
Lung
Adrenal Gland
Divine Gate
Sympathetic Nerve
Internal Secretion

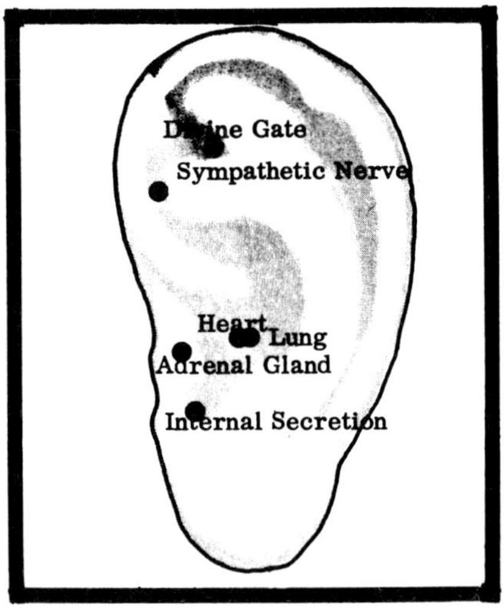

UROLOGICAL SYSTEM

Examples: Frequent micturition (frequent urination), enuresis (bed-wetting), cystitis (inflammation of urinary bladder).

Points: Kidney
Bladder
Adrenal Gland
Occiput
Divine Gate
Sympathetic Nerve
Internal Secretion

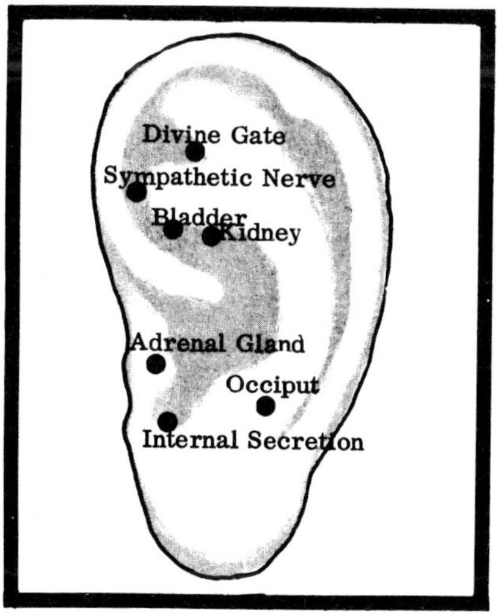

NERVOUS AND MENTAL SYSTEM

Examples: Dizziness, insomnia, dreaminess, migraine headache, trigeminal neuralgia, facial nerve paralysis, intercostal neuralgia, sciatica, neurasthenia, hysteria, heat stroke.

Points: Subcortex
Occiput
Forehead
Heart
Stomach
Kidney
Divine Gate

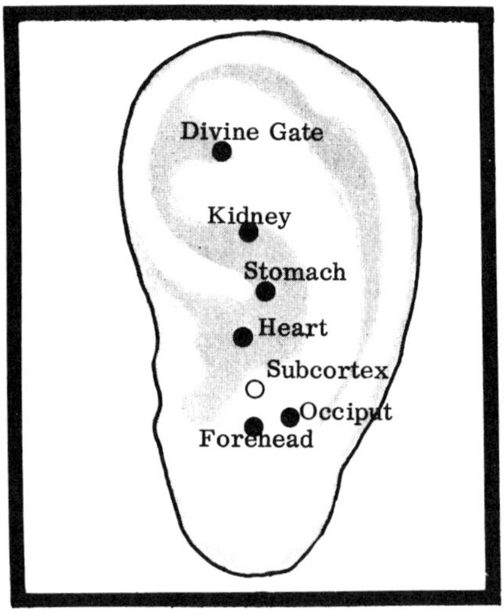

FEMALE DISORDERS

Examples: Dysmenorrhea (painful menstruation), leukorrhea (whitish discharge from vagina), irregular menstruation, menopause, postpartum uteralgia (pain in uterus), prolapse of uterus, inflammation of uterine appendage, external vaginal itching.

Points: Ovary
Internal Secretion
Kidney
Uterus
Sympathetic Nerve

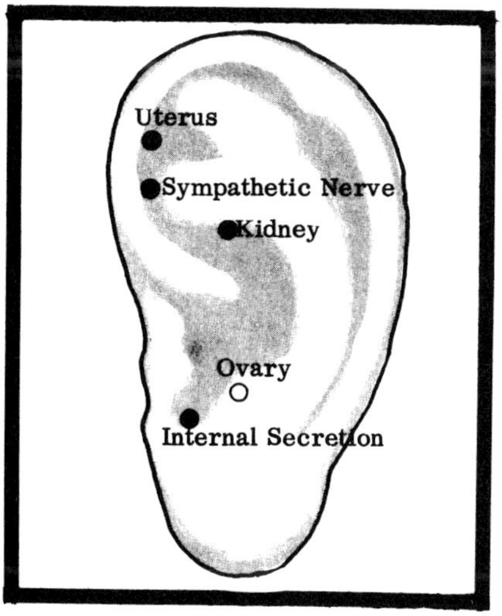

DISORDERS OF THE SENSE ORGANS – EAR

Examples: Otitis media (inflammation of middle ear), tinnitus (ringing in ear), weakening of hearing, Meniere's syndrome (disorder of internal ear characterized by deafness, dizziness and ringing in ear).

Points: Occiput
Kidney
Divine Gate
Internal Ear
External Ear

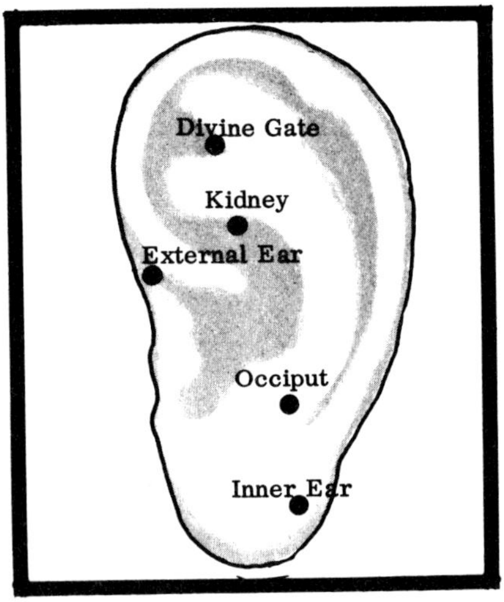

DISORDERS OF THE SENSE ORGANS – NOSE

Examples: Nosebleeding, rhinitis (inflammation of nose), sinusitis.

Points: Internal Nose
Adrenal Gland
Forehead
Lung

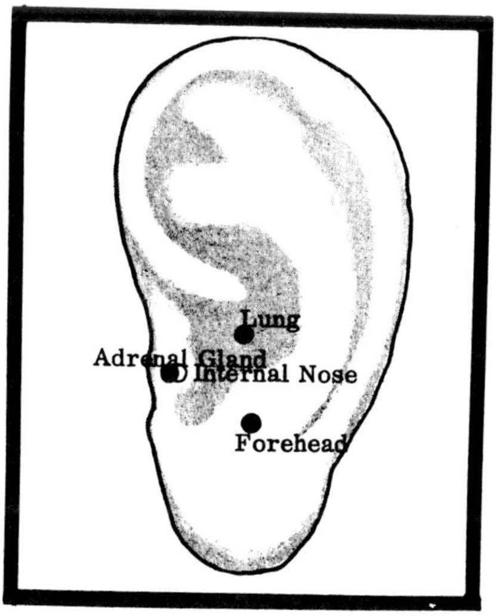

DISORDERS OF THE SENSE ORGANS – MOUTH

Examples: Mouth ulcers, toothache, loose teeth.

Points: Mouth
Upper Jaw
Lower Jaw

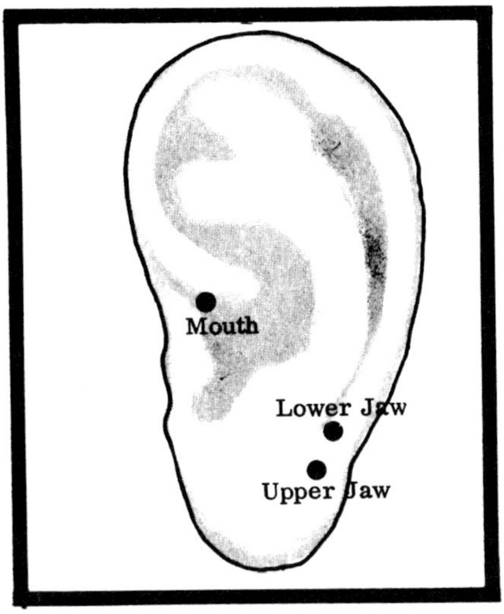

DISORDERS OF THE SENSE ORGANS – EYE

Examples: Conjunctivitis (inflammation of conjunctiva), night blindness, double vision, glaucoma, nearsightedness.

Points: Eye
Liver
Spleen
Eye 1
Eye 2

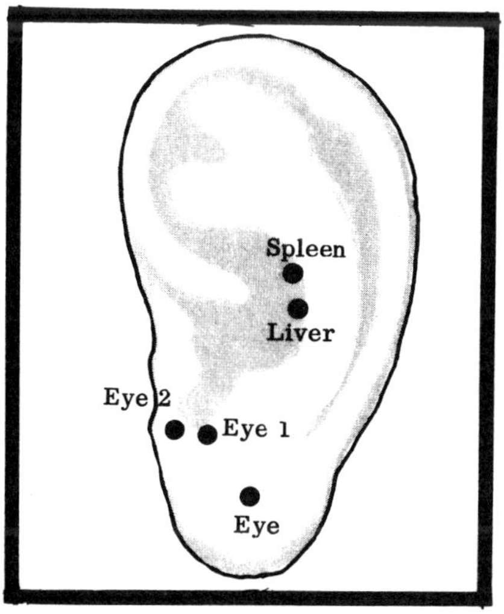

DISORDERS OF THE SENSE ORGANS – SKIN

Examples: Inflammation of skin follicle, shingles, itching, urticaria (skin condition characterized by appearance of intensely itching wheals or welts with elevated, usually white, centers surrounded by areas of redness), dermatitis, prickly heat, hair loss, baldness, acne, eczema, skin rash.

Points: Lung
Occiput
Internal Secretion
Adrenal Gland
Divine Gate

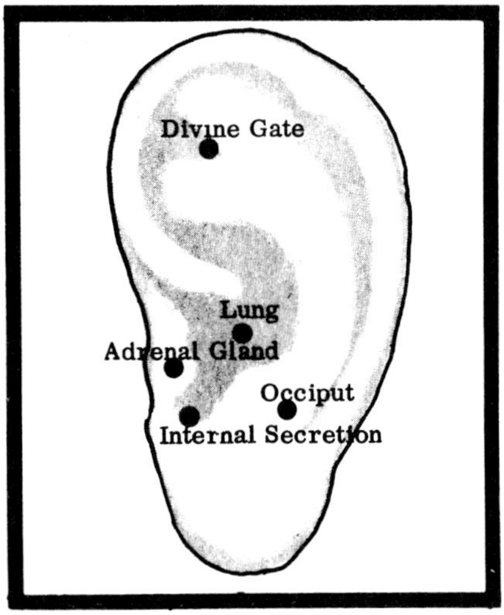

TREATMENT OF OBESITY AND OTHER COMPULSIVE/ADDICTIVE DISORDERS

This chapter discusses treatment of obesity, excessive smoking, drug addiction, alcoholism and hangover due to alcohol. Effective treatment of these disorders by ear acupuncture grew out of research in medical schools and treatment centers. Its popularity has captured the imagination of Americans across the nation. A number of papers have been published in scientific journals reporting the effectiveness of acupuncture in obesity, smoking, alcoholism and drug addiction. Research studies are very encouraging.

OBESITY

Points: Stomach, Mouth, Hunger, and Divine Gate.

Technique

First locate the most responsive point(s) among the first three points of both ears: Stomach, Mouth, and Hunger. Then apply fingernail massage over that particular point(s). If you don't find a point which is more responsive than others, fingernail massage each of them. Place your thumb or one of your fingers at the back of the ear to aid the massage. Massage hard and as fast as you can to produce strong stimulation to reduce your appetite. Mild or weak manipulation may increase appetite.

Massage one point at a time for a minute or two. The best time to do it is half an hour before each meal, or whenever you feel hungry. Massage the points at least three times daily.

Use finger tip to massage lightly the Divine Gate. This point may be massaged on one or both ears, depending on responsiveness in each ear. You may massage this point at any time. This point, when stimulated, helps keep you in good spirit and balance.

On the average, you may expect to lose two to five pounds per week if you are doing it regularly and properly. You may continue to use this technique as long as you want to continue to lose weight. However, results are more encouraging in the first few weeks. If, after reaching desired weight level, you find that you are regaining weight, you may

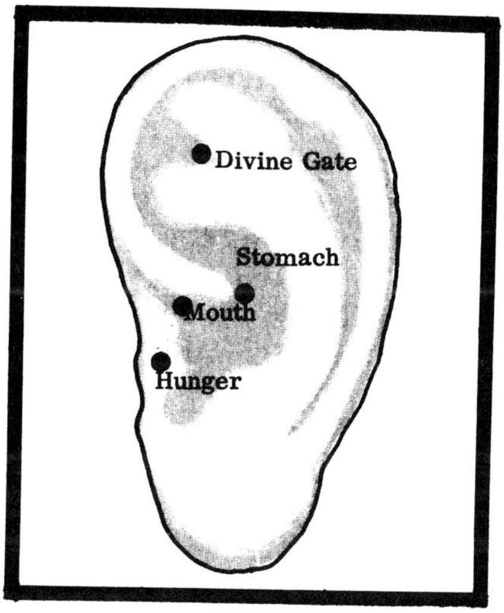

maintain a preventive measure against gaining weight by repeating finger nail massage whenever necessary.

Diet

Proper dieting is an excellent aid for a weight control program. Please consult your physician or a nutritionist for your own menus. Presented here is a list of some DO's and DON'T's for your diet:

DOs:
1. Eat only when you are hungry.
2. Eat slowly and chew thoroughly.
3. Eat *fresh*, natural foods and *fresh* juices.

DON'Ts:
1. No fluid intake with your meal. If you want to drink, do so at least 15 minutes before the meal. Drinking at mealtime may increase your appetite.

2. Avoid canned food, processed foods or drink.
3. Try to avoid intake of salt, sugar, sweets. Salt contributes to holding water; sweets contain carbohydrates and are high in calories.
4. Stay away from high carbohydrates, fatty dairy products.
5. Eat less bread, potatoes, cereals, carrots.
6. Do not snack between meals.
7. Do not use stimulants such as alcohol, or coffee.

Remarks

Finger massage does not take away your weight. It reduces your appetite and cuts your habit of excessive eating. And it accomplishes this without your feeling hungry. The author has heard good reports from patients: "I am eating less, and yet I feel full." "I find the food tasting better. I am eating only half of what I used to." "I feel better about myself."

Self-motivation is very important. Think positively and want to lose weight. Massage of the ear points will remind you.

Exercise cannot be forgotten. This is by far the most natural way to lose weight.

SMOKING (AND DRUG ADDICTION)

Points: Lung, Divine Gate

Technique

The Lung point actually covers a large area. Therefore, you must be very careful to detect the right point. Use a finger nail to massage this point with hard pressure and do it fast. Do this several times daily or whenever the craving starts.

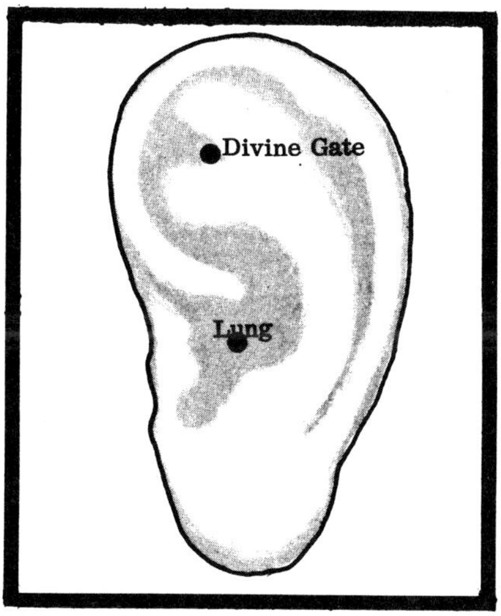

Diet

Do you want to stop smoking? How about fasting for two days? You may take some fresh vegetable juice during your fast. A fast will help clean out the nicotine in the digestive system, especially the bowels.

Remarks

Most patients respond well to this treatment. However, it is difficult to cut off the habit completely. If you are smoking from 20 to 50 cigarettes per day, you may expect to reduce the amount to one or two per day.

For drug addiction, it only provides symptomatic relief of withdrawal (stomach cramps, vomiting, sweating, running nose, etc.). However, if used continuously, it has been reported that the craving for drugs can be alleviated.

In 1972, the first study of treatment of drug addiction by ear acupuncture was reported by Drs. H. L. Wen and Y. C. Cheung from Kwong Wah Hospital, Hong Kong. In that study, 40 cases of addicts (30 opium and 10 heroin) were treated. Preliminary results showed that 39 were discharged and were free of drug addiction. However, 10 received more treatments after discharge. All experienced a sense of general well-being.

In another recent study on animals by the National Institute of Drug Abuse, Dr. Lorenz Ng, et al., reported that stimulation of the ear in morphine-implanted rats could reduce rat activity such as teeth chattering and "wet dog" shakes. This study provides an experimental base that ear stimulation can alleviate the distress of withdrawal without producing undesirable side effects.

ALCOHOLISM (AND HANGOVER)

Points: Liver, Drunk Point, Divine Gate

Technique

Massage both the Liver and Drunk Points with fingernail. Aid the massage by placing thumb at back of the ear. Massage fast and hard to give strong stimulation. Look carefully for the Liver point; sometimes, it may move to the Lung area. In that case, massage the Lung point.

Massage Divine Gate if not comfortable with this treatment. Massaging Divine Gate will give you a feeling of well-being.

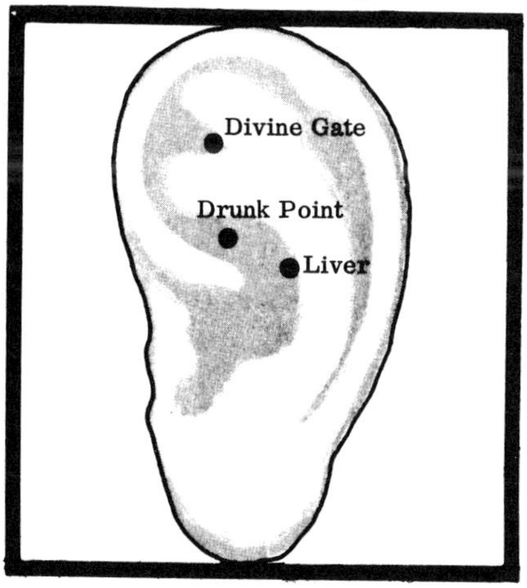

Diet

According to Chinese tradition, American ginseng (generally available in health food stores or herb stores) is excellent in treating alcoholism or hangover. Simply make tea from it or chew it.

TREATMENT OF PAIN SYNDROMES

Treatment of pain syndromes by ear stimulation has proven effective. It is especially good for pain due to sprains, inflammation, neuralgia, arthritis, etc. In a study at the University Hospital, Pain Clinic, London, Canada, ear acupuncture was used on 27 patients with pain from various problems. Results indicated that relief of pain was immediate in 25 patients. In some patients, pain was completely abolished; others reported modification of pain.

GENERAL POINTS FOR PAIN RELIEF

Points: Divine Gate, Subcortex, Adrenal Gland.

Technique

Above points are excellent for relief of pain and/or inflammation. Any one or all of these points can be used for pain felt anywhere in the body. Then add the corresponding point as pain occurs in that part of the body — that is, if pain is in the elbow, add ear point Elbow; if pain is in the wrist, add ear point Wrist.

Generally, points are chosen in the ear corresponding to side on which pain is felt. If pain is central or on both sides, use points in both ears.

Apply hard fingernail pressure if pain is severe. If not, use a finger tip or flat.

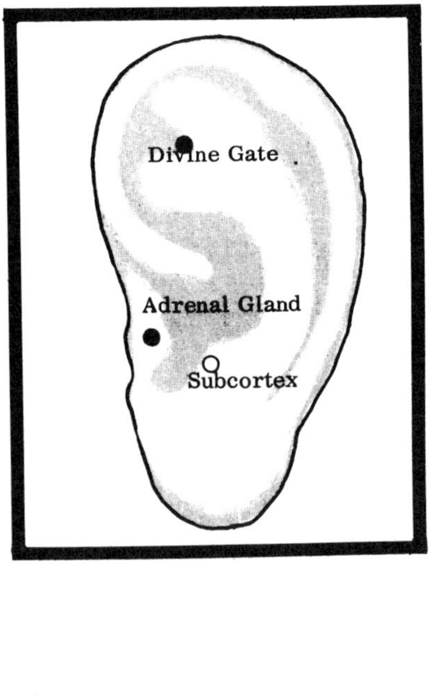

Diet

When patients are in pain, the following foods are forbidden:

1. Iced food or drink.
2. Sour foods such as vinegar, pickle, lemon, pineapple, etc.
3. Alcoholic drinks.
4. Irritating foods such as pepper, hot sauce or spices.
5. Seafood with shells such as lobster, shrimp or crab.

Remarks

Relief of pain by ear acupressure is only symptomatic. It may not take care of the cause of the disorder. If problem persists, consult a physician immediately.

Note: To receive the most beneficial effect, it is necessary to move the painful area of the body while giving treatment. Details of type of movement are described for each case.

FACIAL REGION

Point: Cheek

Technique

While you massage the Cheek point, open and close your mouth in order to produce movement of the facial region. Do it slowly and carefully. If the movement creates severe pain, don't over-stimulate.

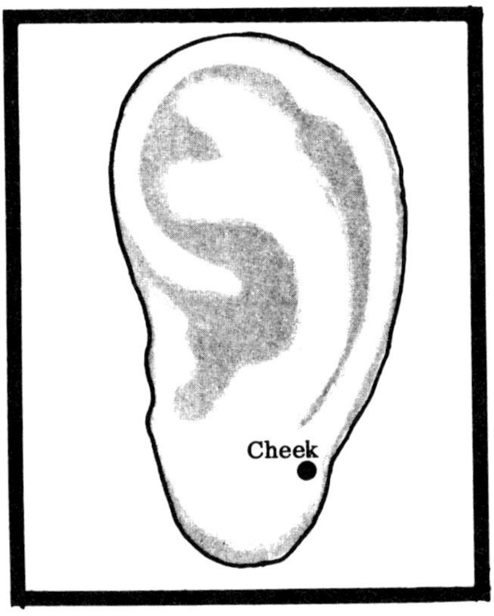

NECK

Point: Neck

Technique

Even if there is no pain in the neck, this point is always responsive, because it also responds to tension and stiffness of the neck. It is astonishing to find that we have tension all the time. In 8 out of 10 cases, this point is responsive.

Massage it in a sitting position, and move your head (without moving your body) from right to left, from left to right, up and down, and down and up. Do it slowly and carefully.

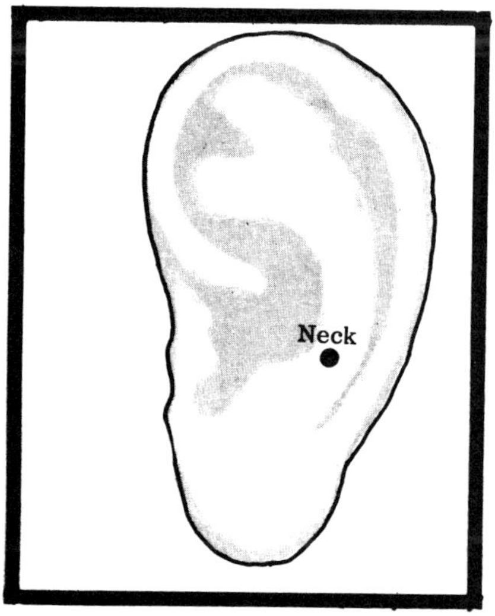

TOOTHACHE

Points: Upper Jaw, Lower Jaw, Divine Gate, Toothache, Throat-Tooth.

Technique

Find the most sensitive, responsive point among the above, and massage it.

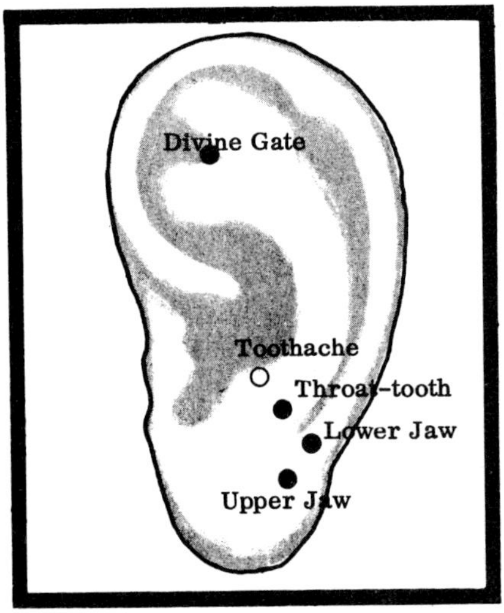

SHOULDER

Point: Shoulder

Technique

While you massage the Shoulder point, move your arm slowly in a circular motion.

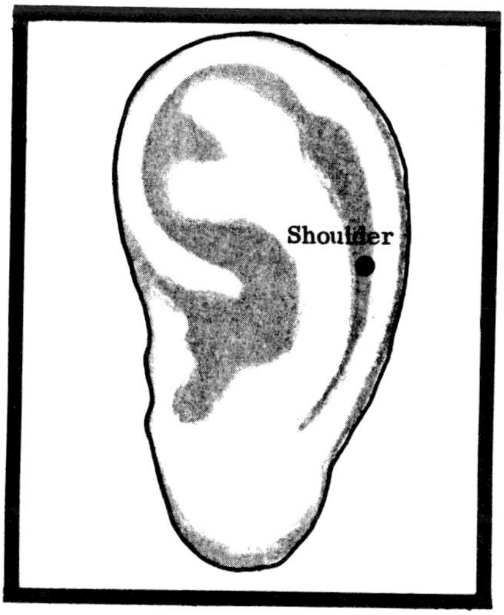

ELBOW

Point: Elbow

Technique

Massage above point and move your forearm to and away from your body.

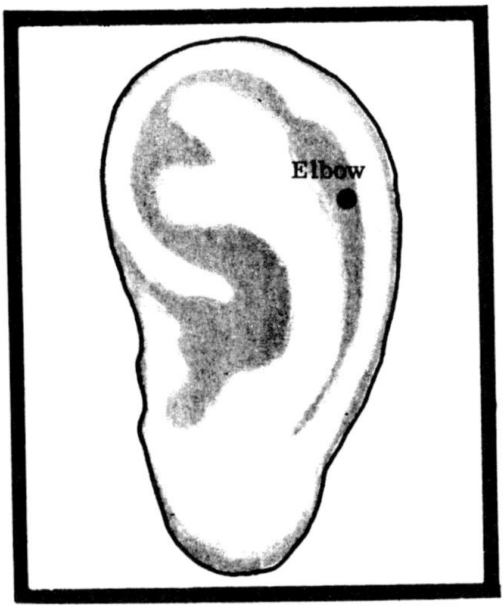

WRIST

Point: Wrist

Technique

Locate the Wrist point and massage it. Move your wrist in a circular motion.

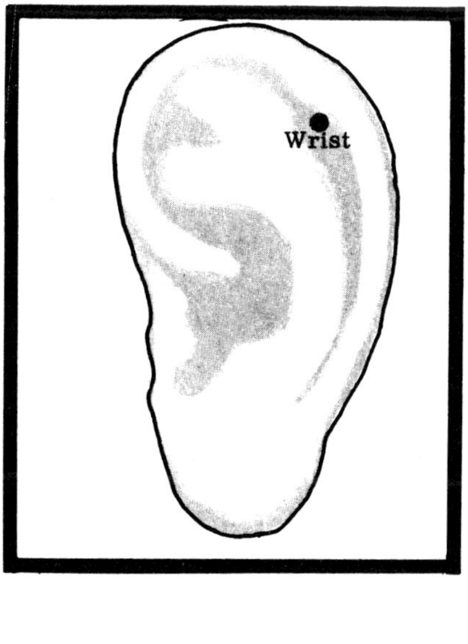

FINGER

Point: Finger

Technique

Massage the point while opening and closing your hand. Do it slowly.

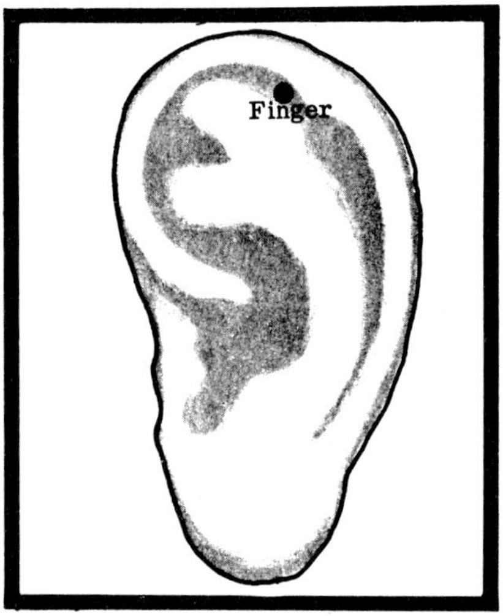

SPINAL COLUMN

Points: Cervical Vertebrae, Thoracic Vertebrae, Lumbar Vertebrae, Sacral Vertebrae.

Technique

First determine the location of pain in the spine, then massage the corresponding point. While you massage the point, bend yourself forward, backward, and sideward. Do this very carefully and slowly. If you cannot move at all, don't proceed.

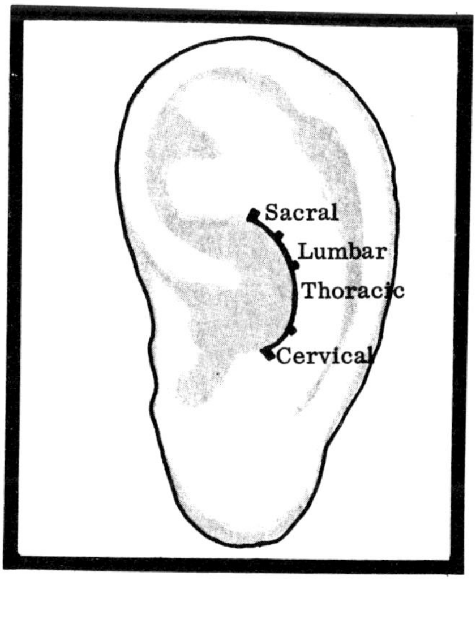

LOW BACK

Point: Lumbago

Technique

Massage the point while in a standing position. Move the lower back forward, sideward and backward.

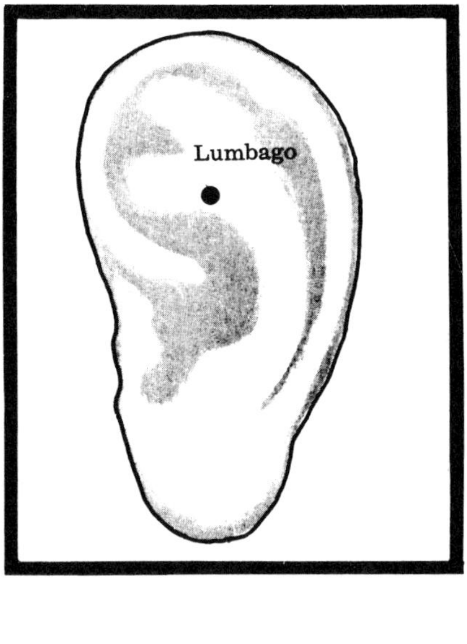

CHEST

Point: Chest

Technique

Massage the point while lying down. Take a deep breath and repeat this several times during the massage.

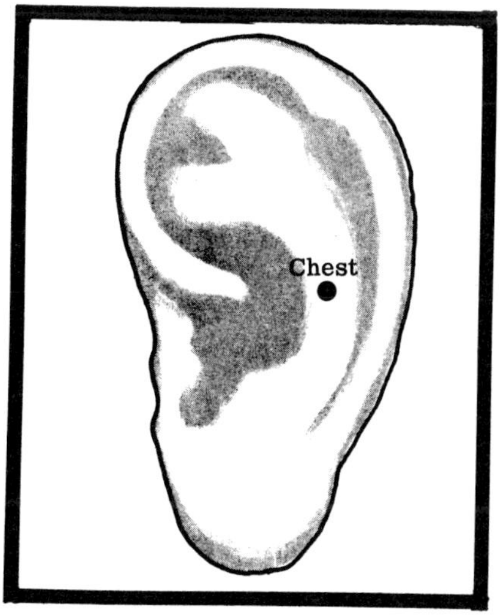

ABDOMEN

Point: Abdomen

Technique

Massage the point and massage the surface over the abdominal area. Lying down will make you more comfortable and relaxed.

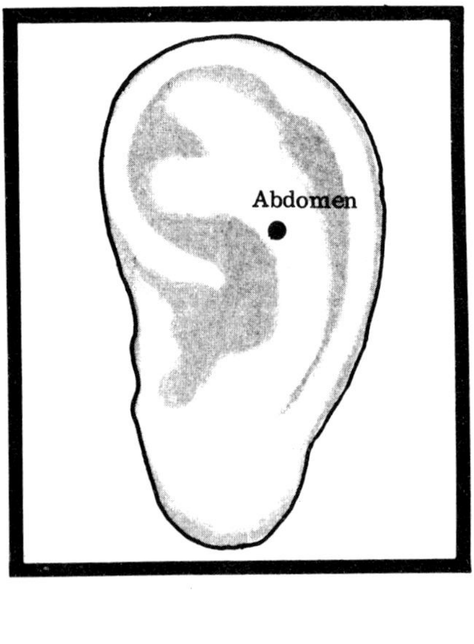

HIP

Point: Hip

Technique

Massage the point while in a standing position. Move the buttock around.

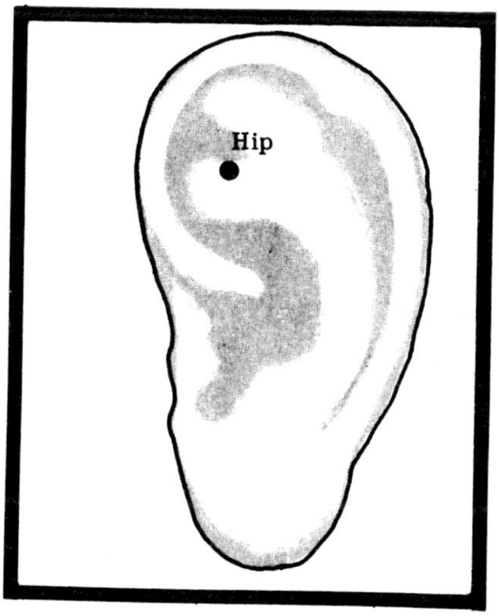

KNEE

Point: Knee

Technique

Massage the point while in a sitting position. Move the knee forward, sideward, backward or in a circular motion.

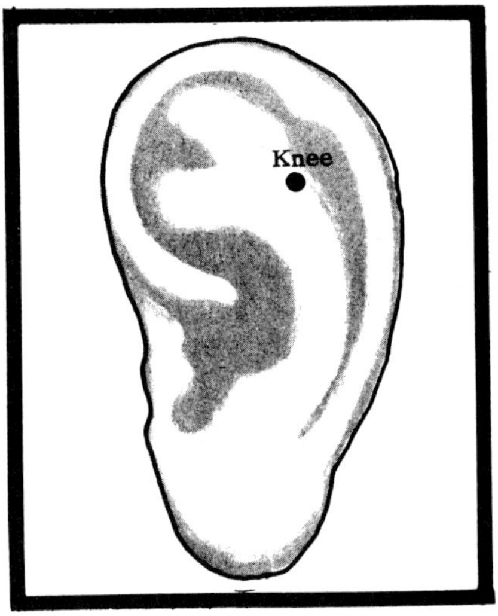

ANKLE

Point: Ankle

Technique

Massage the point while in a sitting or lying position. Move the ankle in a circular motion.

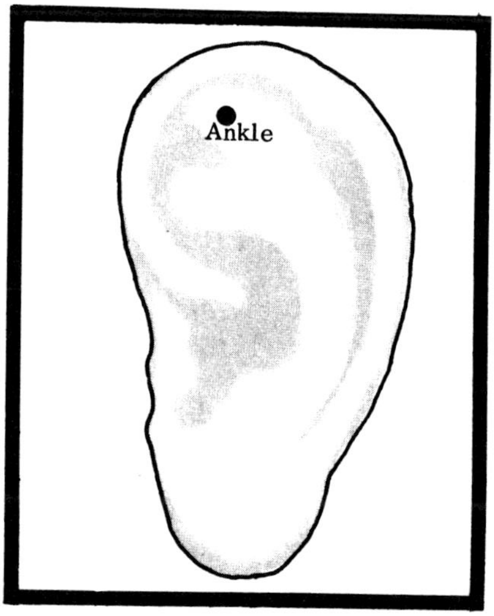

TREATMENT OF HEADACHES

General Technique

Use point(s) as indicated under each type of headache. Massage the point(s) three times a day. The best time to massage it is when you have the headache.

Diet

Follow the same instructions given for pain syndromes.

Remarks

To aid the above technique, it is highly recommended that you massage the body over the two acupuncture points Ho-Ku (Large Intestine 4) and Feng-chih (Gall Bladder 20). These two points have proven very successful for headache treatment.

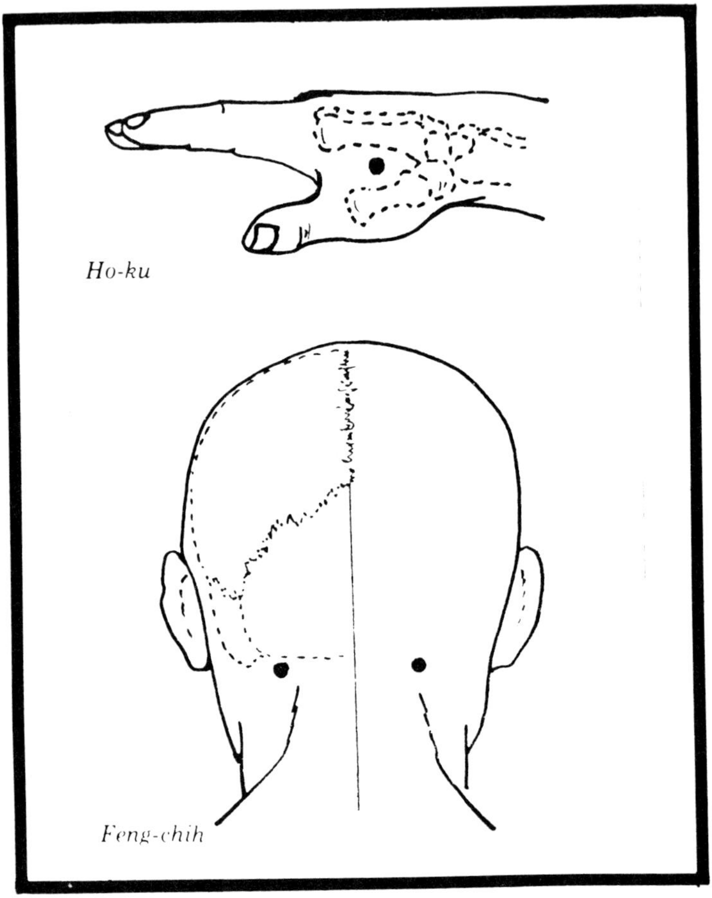
Ho-ku
Feng-chih

FRONTAL HEADACHE

Points: Forehead, Subcortex, Divine Gate

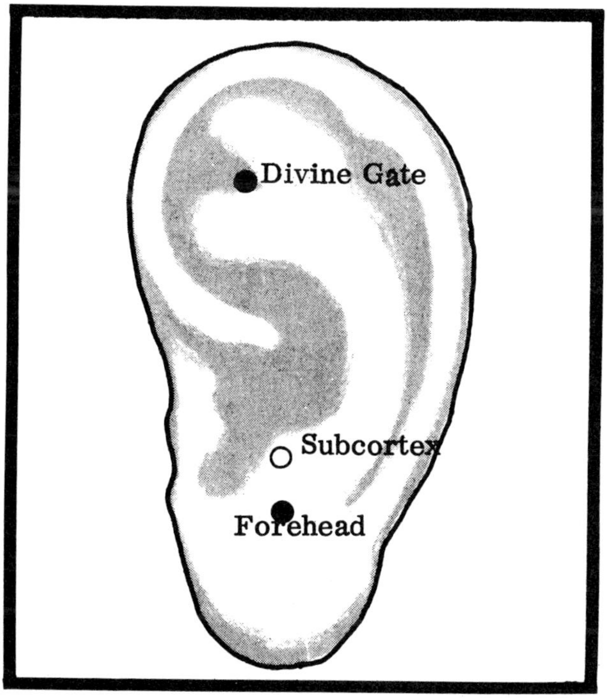

OCCIPITAL

Points: Occiput, Subcortex, Divine Gate

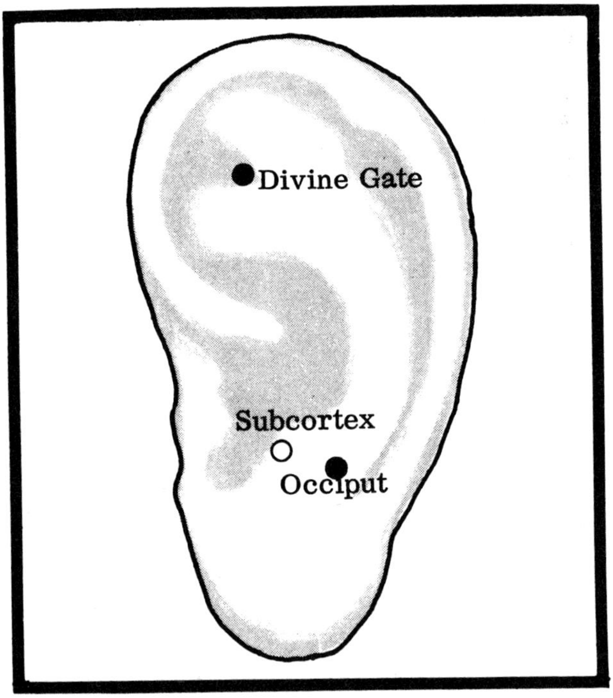

VERTICAL HEADACHE

Points: Vertex, Subcortex, Divine Gate

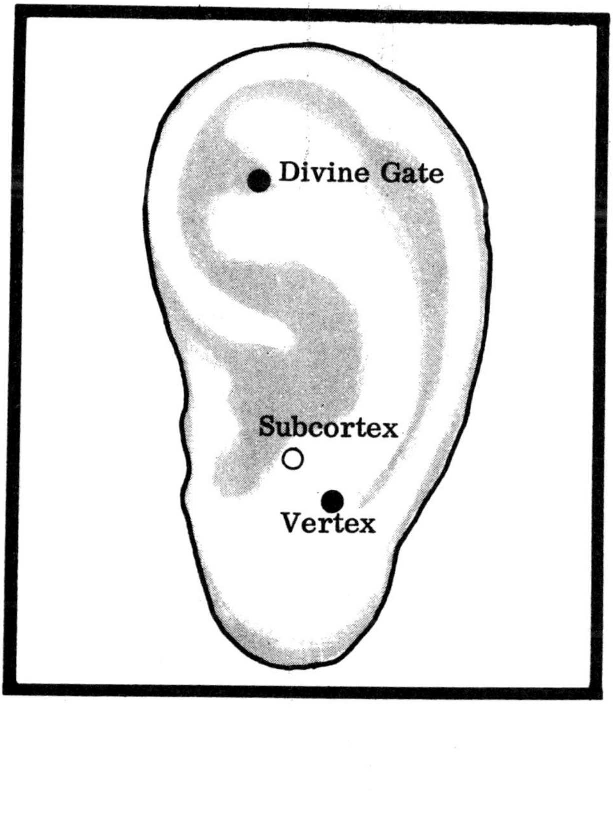

MIGRAINE

Points: Subcortex, Temple, Liver

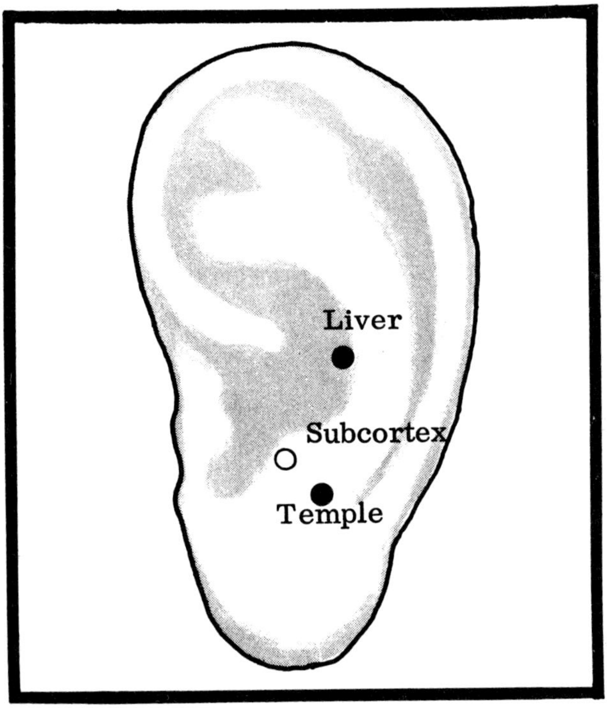

TREATMENT OF REPRODUCTIVE DISORDERS

It may sound ridiculous to treat reproductive disorders in the ear. However, this technique works. Looking at the ear physiology chart up close, you will find there are sex points such as External Genital Organs, Ovary, Testis, etc.

IMPOTENCE

Points: External Genital Organs, Testis, Uterus, Kidney.

Technique

Massage all points. Apply light pressure at least three times a day. Continuous massage for at least three weeks may be required for any results.

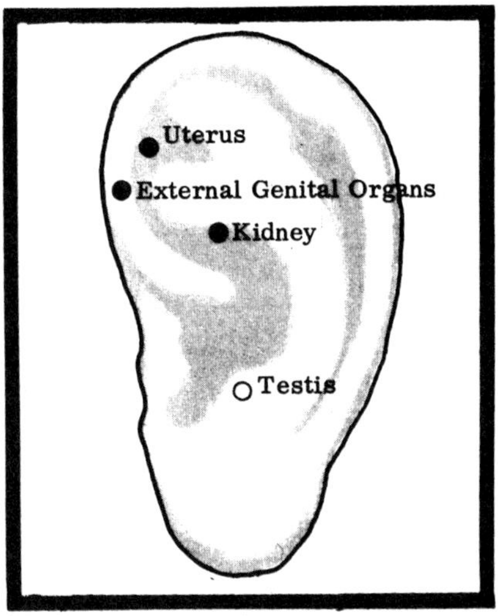

Diet

Pork kidney, squab and lamb are recommended for your diet. Chinese ginseng is also a good herb for energy. You may make soup from it with chicken.

PREMATURE EJACULATION

Points: Uterus, External Genital Organs, Testis, Internal Secretion, Divine Gate.

Technique

Massage only the responsive point(s) of the above points. Apply light pressure three times a day continuously for three weeks.

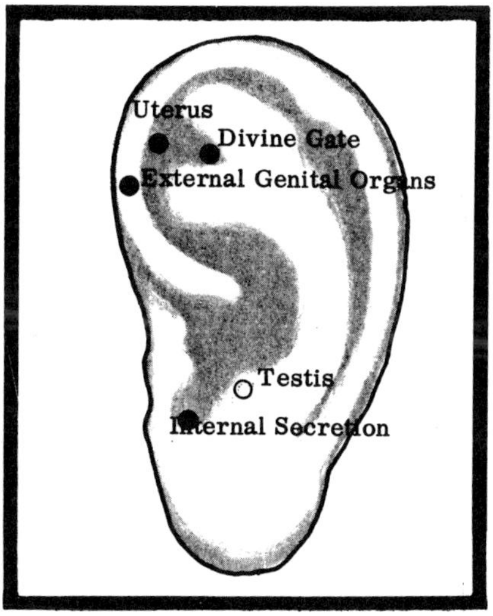

Diet

Same as for impotence.

Remarks

To remain calm before sex, massage Divine Gate. This is a good point for sedation.

PROSTATITIS

Points: Prostate Gland, Internal Secretion, Kidney.

Technique

Massage all points. Continuous massage for at least three weeks is required. Massage three times a day.

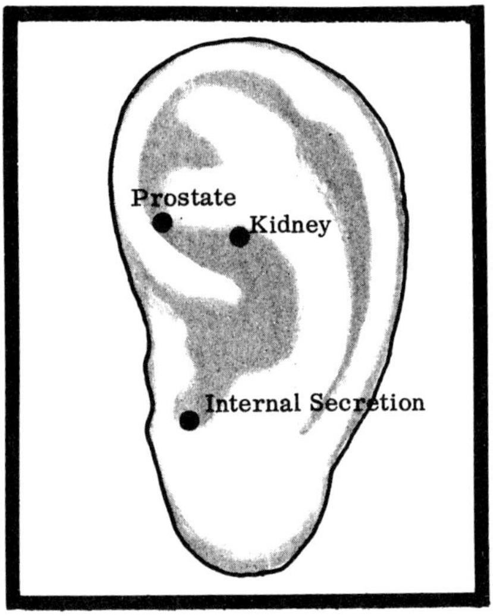

Diet

Stay away from hot food, spices and stimulants. Don't eat or drink just before sleeping.

IRREGULAR MENSES

Points: Uterus, Ovary, Internal Secretion, Kidney.

Technique

Massage only points that are responsive. Do it three times a day for three weeks. Apply light pressure.

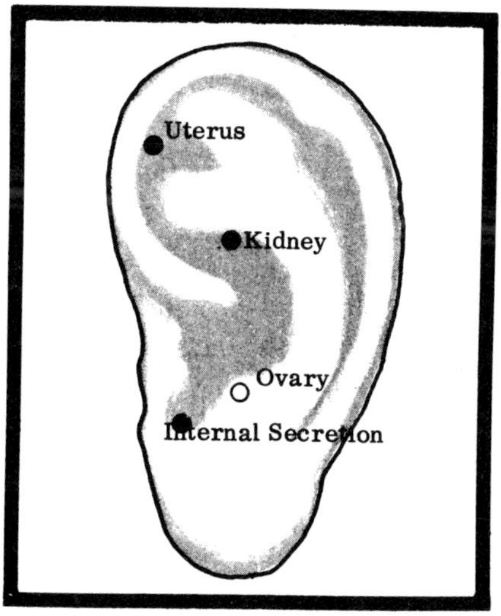

Diet

Do not take any raw or iced food or drink.

MENOPAUSE

Points: Uterus, Ovary, Internal Secretion.

Technique

Massage responsive point(s) only. Do it three times a day for three weeks. Apply light pressure.

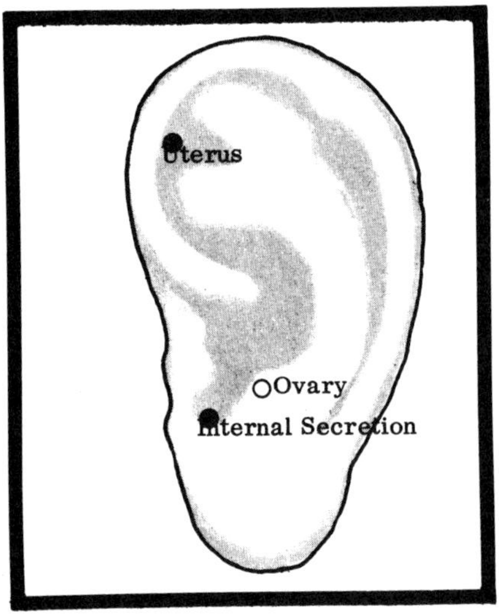

Diet

Do not take any raw or iced food or drink.

PAINFUL MENSTRUATION

Points: Uterus, Sympathetic Nerve, Internal Secretion, Subcortex, Divine Gate.

Technique

Massage points that are responsive. Apply hard pressure for severe pain, light pressure for mild pain.

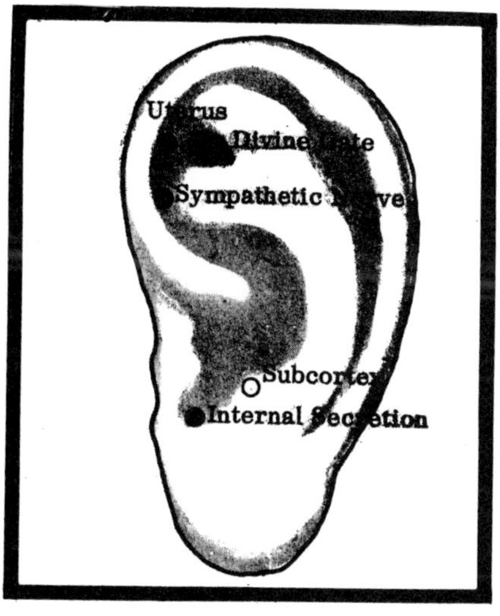

Diet

Follow instructions for pain syndromes. Be sure to stay away from raw or iced food or drink.

OTHER SELECTED CASES
(In Alphabetical Order)

TO ENLARGE THE BREAST

Points: Chest, Mammary Gland, Internal Secretion

NOTE: Technique is rather recent and results preliminary. Patients claim to have a feeling of fullness in the chest area after treatments. Body points around the breast should also be used.

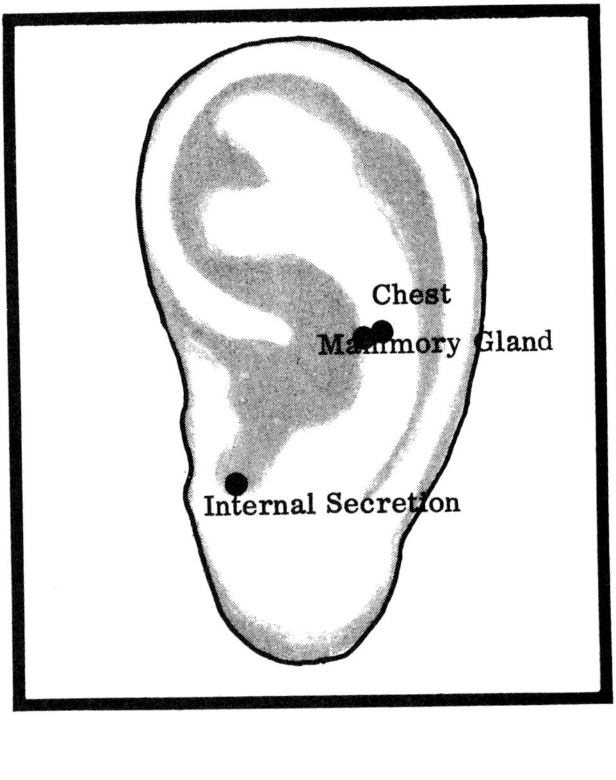

BREATHING DIFFICULTY

Points: Soothing Asthma, Asthma Point, Lung

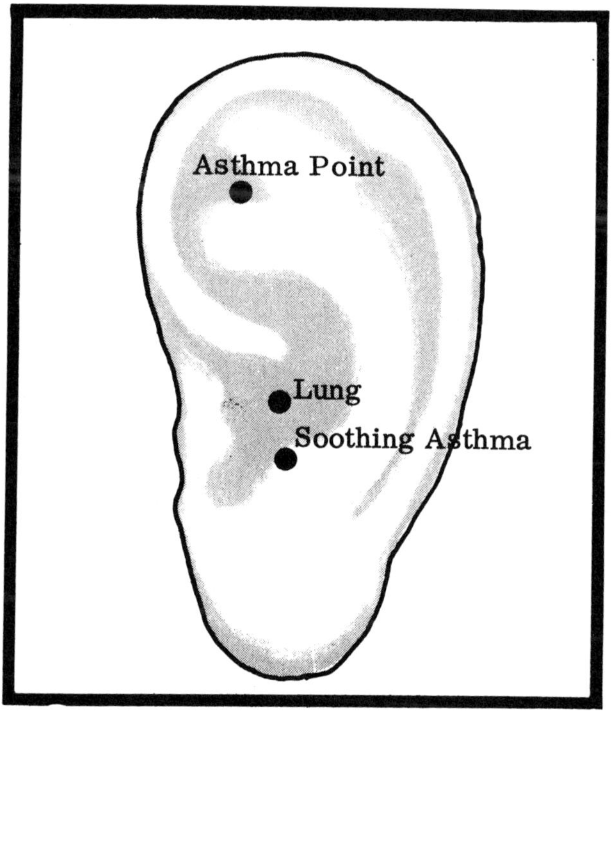

COMMON COLD

Points: Internal Nose, Adrenal Gland, Forehead, Lung

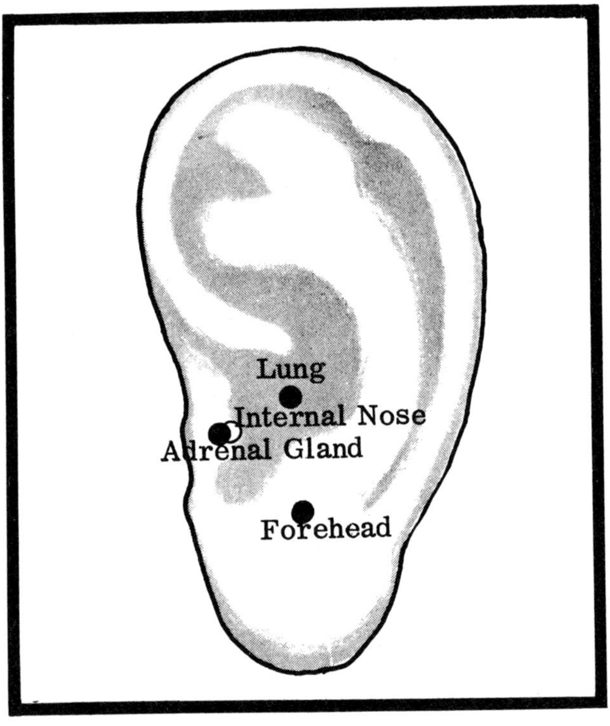

CONSTIPATION

Points: Large Intestine, Lower Section of the Rectum, Subcortex, Constipation.

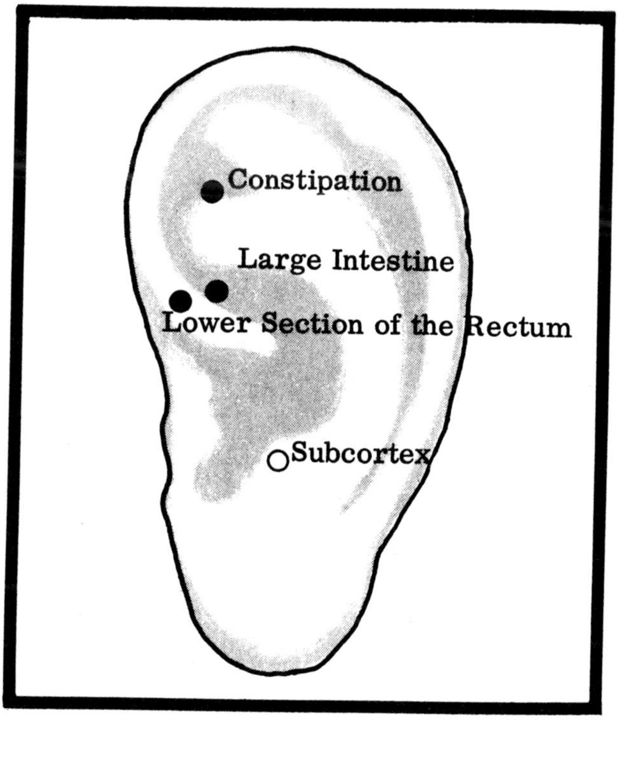

HAIR LOSS

Points: Kidney, Lung, Internal Secretion, Occiput.

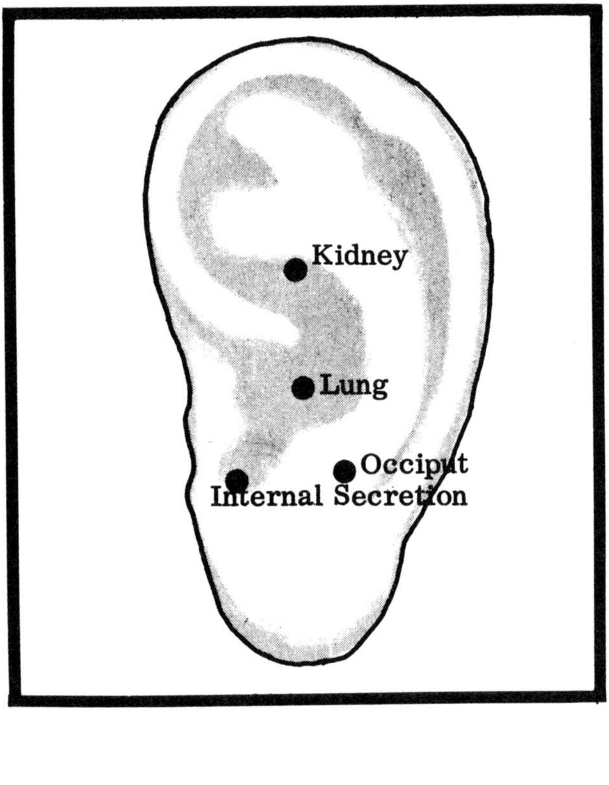

HEMORRHOIDS

Points: Lower Section of the Rectum, Large Intestine, Subcortex, Spleen, Divine Gate.

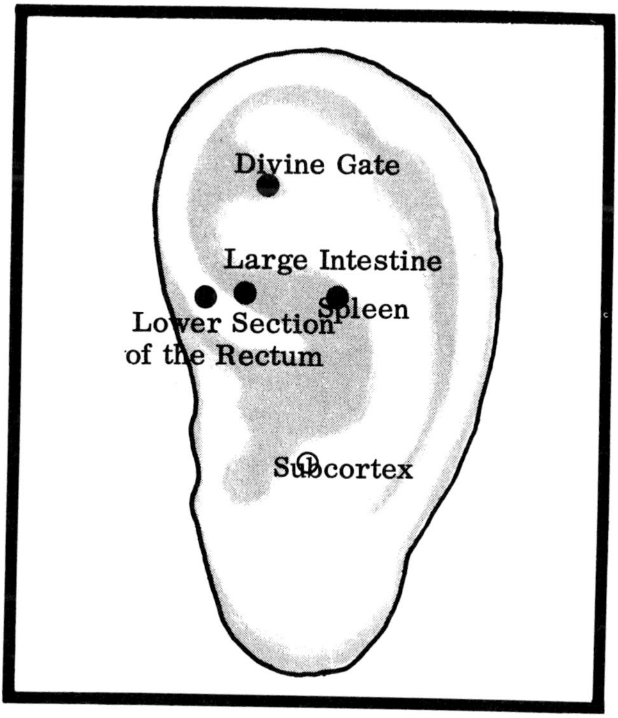

INSOMNIA

Points: Divine Gate, Kidney, Occiput, Heart

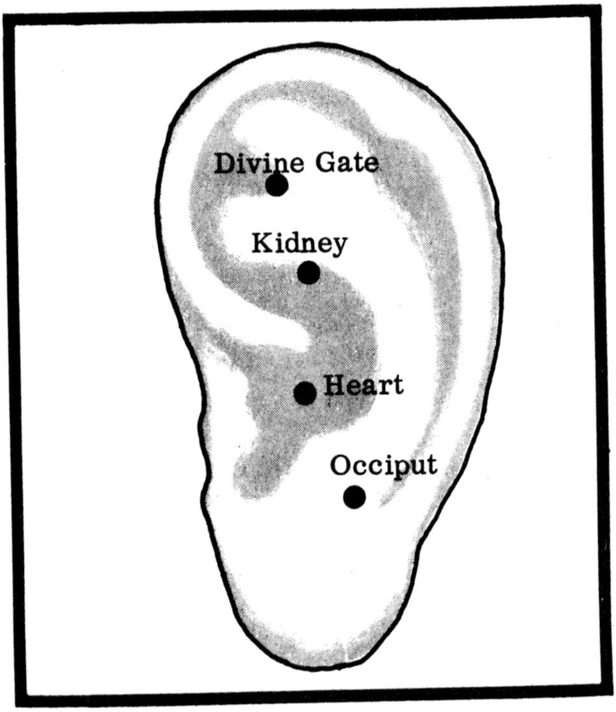

ITCHING

Points: Divine Gate, Lung, Occiput, Internal Secretion, Adrenal Gland, Parotid.

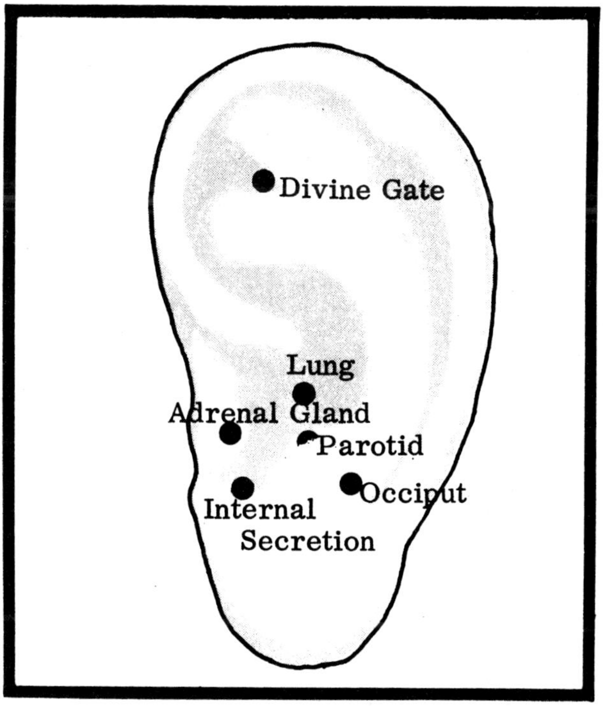

MOTION SICKNESS

Points: Occiput, Stomach, Internal Ear, Divine Gate

NOTE: This technique is also good for prevention.

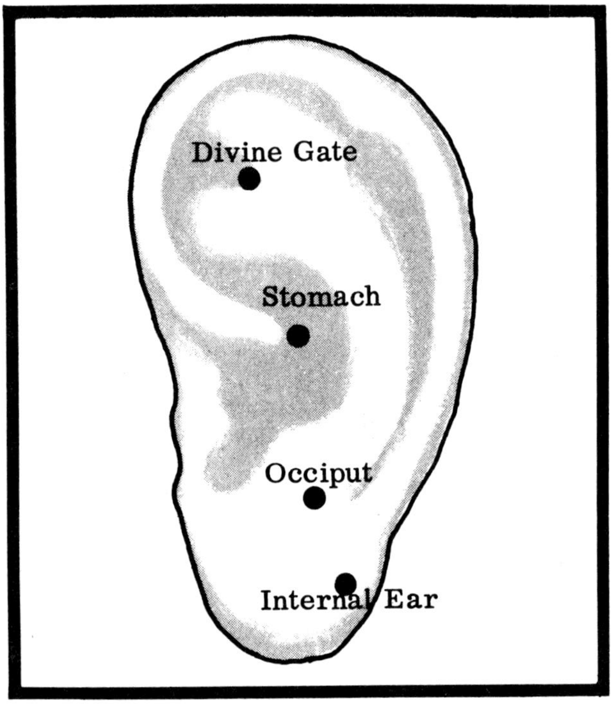

NEURASTHENIA

Points: Kidney, Divine Gate, Occiput, Heart, Stomach, Neurasthenia.

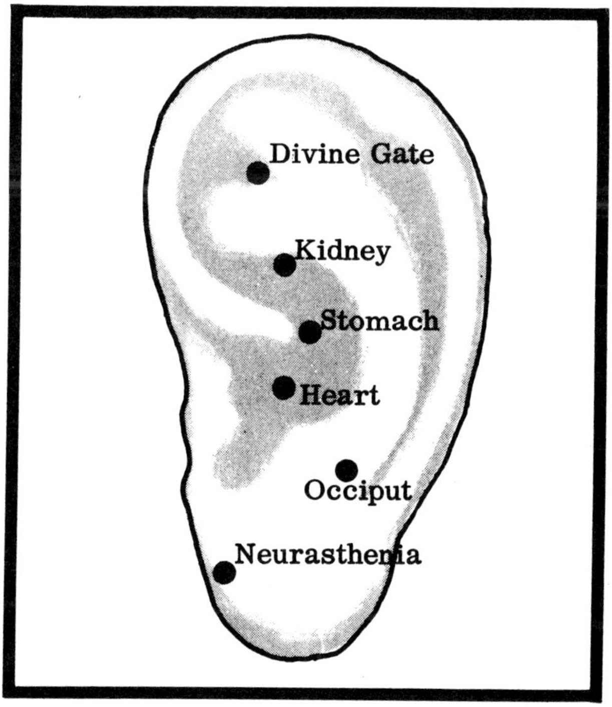

SCIATICA

Points: Sciatic Nerve, Divine Gate

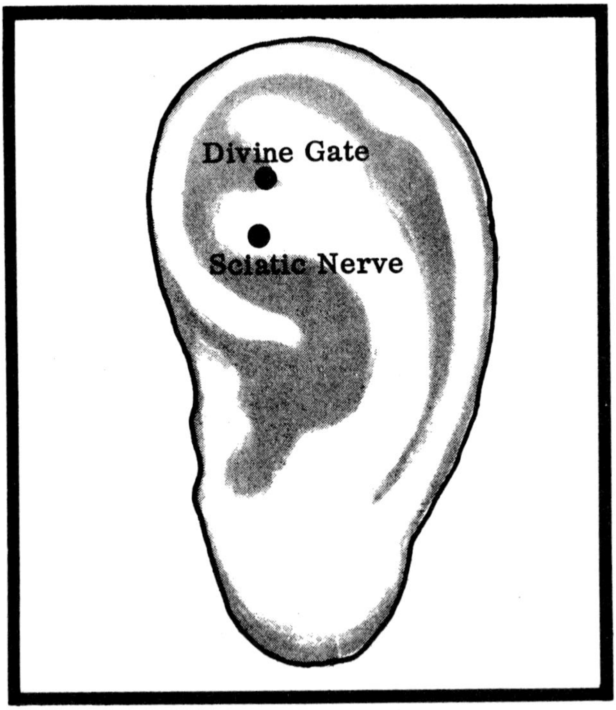

TONSILLITIS

Points: Tonsil 1, 2, 3, 4

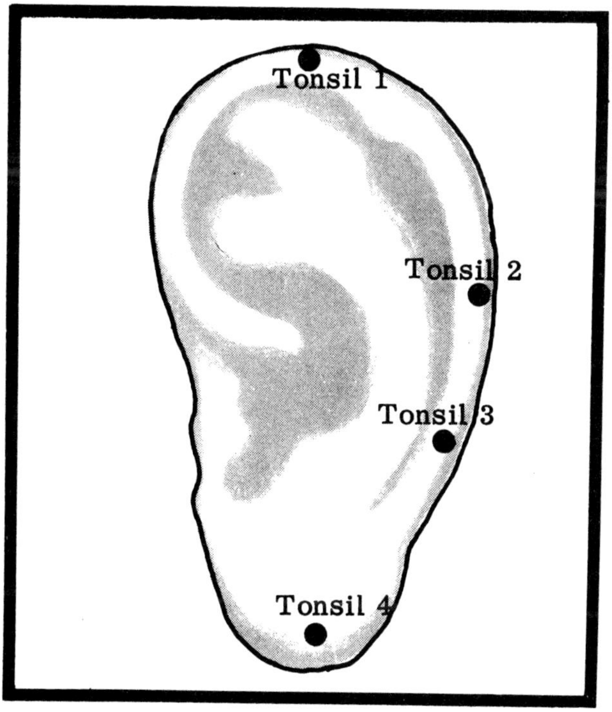

TWISTED NECK

Points: Cervical Disc, Neck, Divine Gate

NOTE: In 9 out of 10 people, the "NECK" point shows a definite response, which means that we suffer some degree of tension and stiffness in the neck area at all times. Therefore, it is always a good exercise to massage the "NECK" point once in awhile.

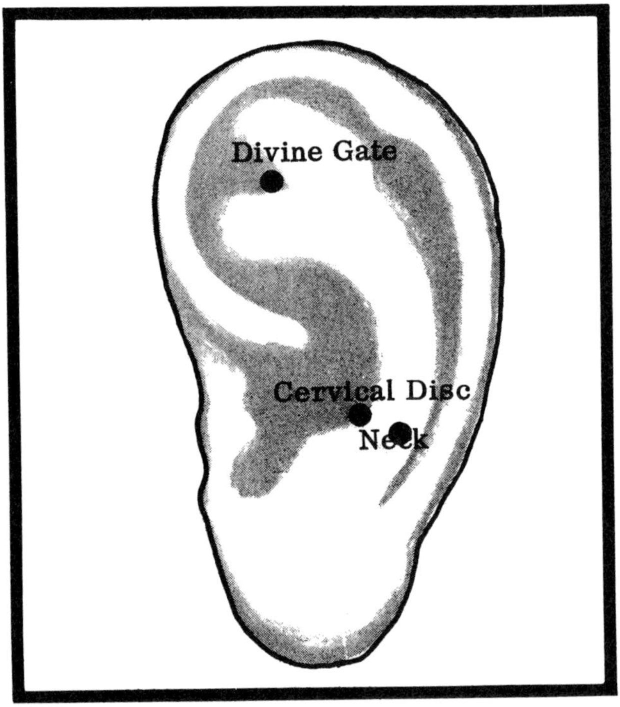

LOSS OF VOICE

Points: Throat, Heart, Lung, Divine Gate, Internal Secretion

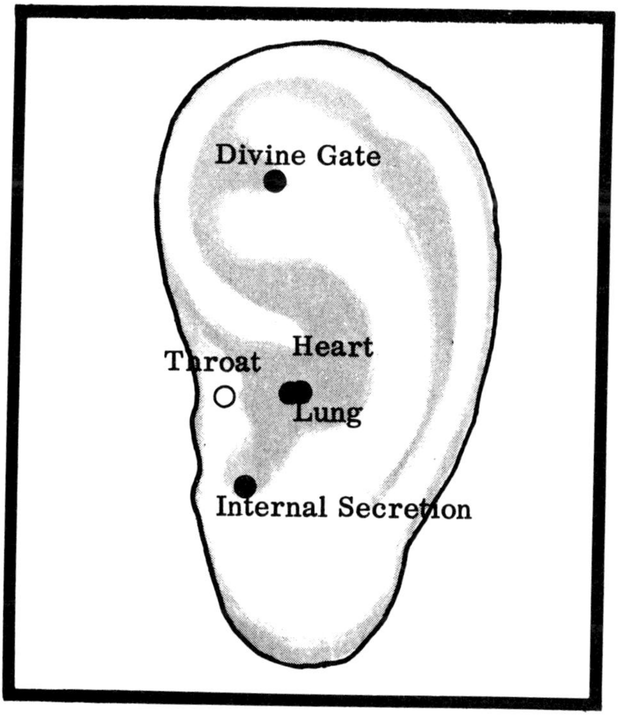

APPENDIX

EAR DIAGNOSIS – Examples:

1) Stomach ulcer – small pimple with red rim in "STOMACH" area.

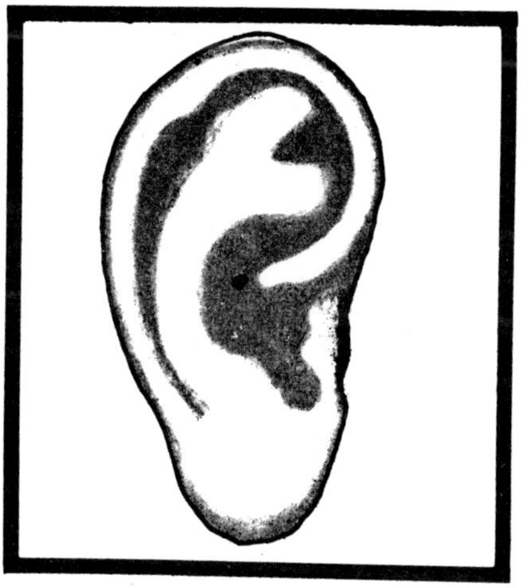

2) Hepatomegalia (enlargement of the liver) – swelling in "LIVER" area.

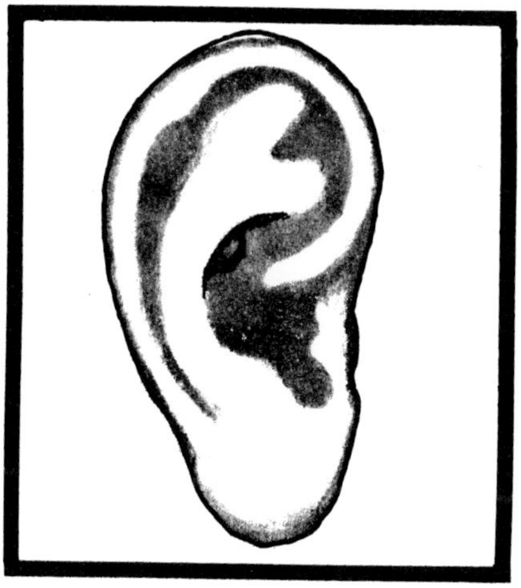

3) Skin Disease – skin peeling in "LUNG" area.

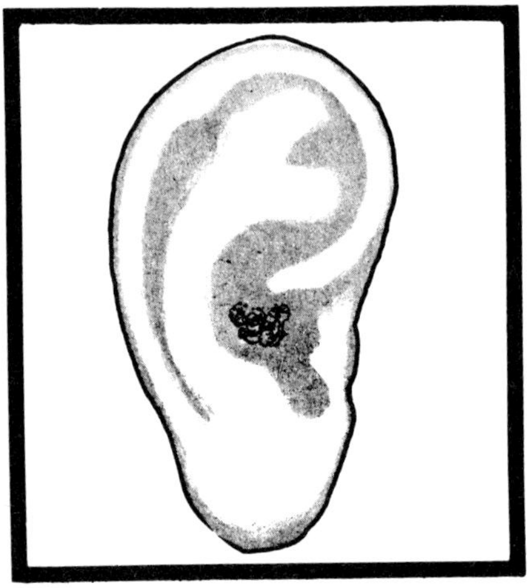

4) Female disease – hives or skin peeling in "UTERUS" area.

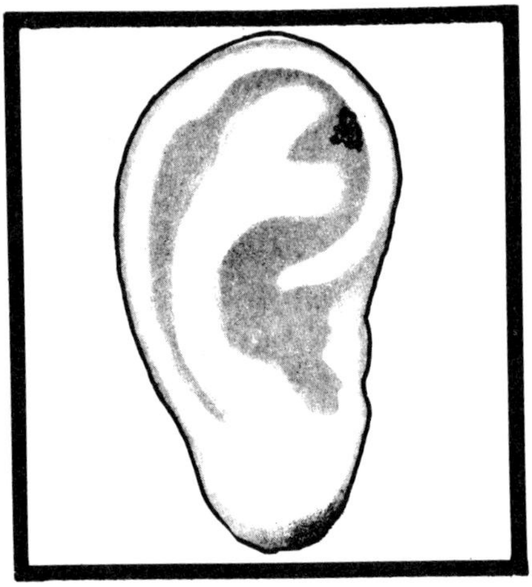

Other recommended books . . .

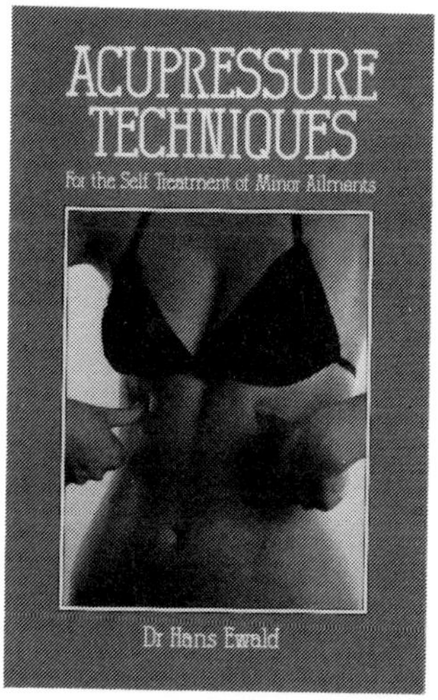

ACUPRESSURE TECHNIQUES

FOR THE SELF-TREATMENT OF MINOR AILMENTS

The techniques of acupressure are easy to understand and anyone can put them to effective use in dealing with discomfort. In this fully illustrated book these techniques, developed from the five thousand year old Chinese healing system of acupuncture, are clearly explained so that you can immediately locate the pressure points and treat yourself. No needles are used, just finger and thumb pressure, and by this method pain can be relieved, the period of many ailments shortened and malfunctions put right. Also the effects of stress, anxiety and tension can be dissipated.

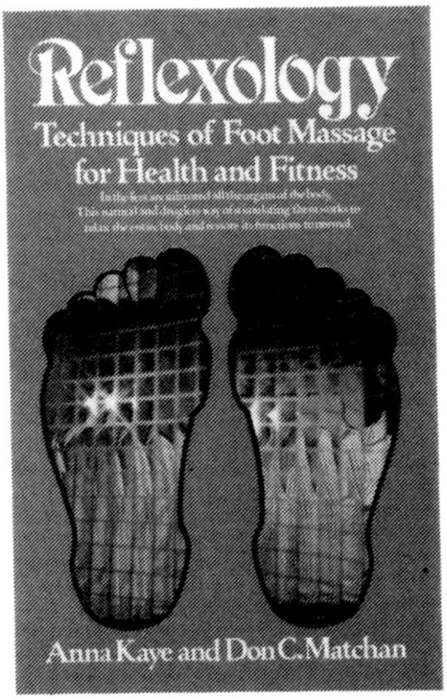

REFLEXOLOGY

THE TECHNIQUES OF FOOT MASSAGE FOR HEALTH AND FITNESS

Anna Kaye & Don Matchan. *Illustrated.* Explains techniques of foot massage, the natural way of stimulating internal organs for restoring body functions to normal. This is an ancient art, used by the Chinese for more than 5,000 years. It is practised primarily on the feet because *in the feet are mirrored all organs of the body.* Treatment details given for allergies, arthritis, asthma, colds, constipation, diabetes, digestive troubles, emphysema, headache, high blood-pressure, muscle cramps, varicose veins, weight problems, hot flushes, etc. Includes chart showing locations of the reflexes and a chapter on American Indian massage.